FUEL YOUR *family*

A CLEAN EATING FAMILY COOKBOOK

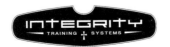

Forward –

Each of my books were birthed from a situation. I didn't sit down and say I'm writing a book today. My first book came from a consistent blog I worked on for over a year. I kept getting requests to save all of the messages into a book to help keep folks on track. My second book happened when I was down for 2 days with Strep throat. It hit me like a ton of bricks. I was so sick and absolutely hated that I couldn't go to work. I reached out to clients and trainers and asked if they would provide a healthy recipe they would feed their family for the holidays. My third book came from my clients needing more ideas on how to take basic ingredients and make them taste great.

This is my 4th book. This one happened the first week of school for Sophie. They took her snack away in 1st grade. She has breakfast at 7am and was expected to go until lunch without a snack. This really surprised me. I know how important it is to fuel a child properly for focus and performance. Sure enough Sophie came home that first week saying she fell asleep 2 days in a row during reading time. This is not good. I don't want my 1st grader falling asleep in class. I decided to create a clean protein muffin for her. I had her help me. Something to provide her with protein, good fat and quality low sugar carbs. This worked. She felt great.

I kept experimenting with different recipes and came up with several versions. We started using different pans to make them more interesting looking. I even turned one of them into an elephant and a flower. She loved it. So far we've shared the recipes with many people and everyone really loves them. This is great food to eat on the go, to fuel your family and feel great.

People often use kids as the excuse for why they cannot eat clean but they truly need to be the reason for why they eat clean. We lead them. If we lead them to garbage they will feel like garbage and perform like garbage. We cannot expect the school system to do it for us. Even in a private school Sophie is offered sugar often. It's an easy reward for a job well done. Sophie doesn't need this. She appreciates the praise, a hug, a sticker or new eraser. Feeding kids sugar daily slows them down and destroys their focus.

These recipes are great options to fuel your family with. This is what we feed Sophie. We have no issues in keeping her happy, fueled and feeling great. She has struggled with abdominal inflammation, intestinal bacteria, allergies and mucus since she was very little. Even at 2 years old she had a hard, distended belly. We took her to Dr. Anna Bone at a very young age for a homeopathic natural approach to her health. We've given Sophie a gluten-free diet with minimal dairy. We avoid corn and soy as well as have minimal sugar. She has 1 off meal a week and she enjoys it with us and looks forward to it.

Some people might say "Won't you create an eating disorder by restricting her?" I say "Won't you create diabetes, SIBO, asthma, chronic sinusitis, irritable bowel syndrome and so on if you don't restrict your kid?" It's all in your approach. We've explained the science to Sophie. She has experienced it for herself. 1 day of off meals with friends including all sorts of junk food had her in so much pain she may never forget it. She knows what happens when she eats healthy and she knows what happens when she eats junk. She knows so much that she has no problem and gives us no issue with it. She enjoys the food we give her. I'm sure she would enjoy a bunch of junk food as well. She respects the why behind what we do. Teach your kids the why. You are the only education for a healthy life they may ever get. My parents always explained why we ate what we ate. I watched my Dad eat healthy my entire life and always knew it was part of why he felt as well as he did and performed as well as he did.

Giving your child a chance at a healthy lifestyle at a young age is a great blessing. The next time you say "I can't eat clean because I have kids" try to turn that around and make it "I must eat clean because I have kids." Eating clean does not have to mean eating plain. Enjoy these recipes. Honor God with the choices you make with your food and the food for your family. God bless you as you fuel your family.

About the Author -

I am the owner of Integrity Training Systems. Serving God through my passion for helping people achieve optimal health.

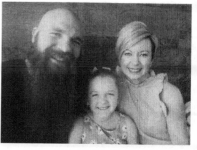

Christ is my focus and serving his purpose. I'm engaged to a Giant Viking, John Morris, and we take care of his daughter Sophie who is 6. She's been part of my life for 4.5 years so I have always considered her my daughter. She is a wonderful blessing that God has given me. Her spirit is amazing. She has shown me that faith comes in all ages, shapes and sizes. She's also shown me that my walk matters. Her Dad John started as my greatest pal, I loved working out with him, sharing Bible verses and encouraging each other in faith. One day he asked if he could court me and I said, "Do you mean take me on a date?" He said, "Oh I know I want to marry you, I just need a chance to talk you into wanting to marry me." So that was that. We will be married soon. God willing very soon. He brought the laughter back in me. God gave me them.

I love my dogs. They might as well be children. My dog Cannon is a lab. He is 15 and handsome with a very distinguished gray beard. He's taken me through great struggles. He came to work with me and really provided me the friendship I needed when the world felt like it had turned it's back on me. When my Godfather Freemont, who was my client died, I inherited his dog, Dolly. I always called Freemont my Godfather because outside of the Lord I don't trust many people. I always trusted Freemont and he always trusted me. He drove me around his farm on his 4 wheeler many times and helped me to find peace in simplicity. His dog, Dolly, was his world. I wouldn't trade her for anything. My mom had a heart attack a while back. We started to take care of her 9 year old dog Sammy. She is as sweet as sugar from the cane. What a blessing to have her under my feet every where I go. My mom is doing much better.

My Mom and Dad are my biggest fans. They listen to my radio show every Sunday. Dad works at the gym everyday. Mom walks the dogs so I can work and she spends time with Sophie when I can't. I watch her teach Sophie self discipline the way she taught me. I am clean, orderly, detailed and successful because my Mom taught me to be. She was a very hard worker all my life and still made time for her family. My Dad should wear a cape. He is truly a hero. If I could pick any quality I would want a man to possess, it would be to have my Dad's work ethic, respect for my Mother and love for his children. He is humble, yet strong. Thank you Lord for an amazing support system.

I have an amazing brother and sister, Kim and Bob, who believe in me and always cheer me on. They make me laugh and fuel me when they tell me they are proud of me. I don't do it for the praise but they matter to me. I love each of them so much.

Integrity Training Systems is my gym in Winghaven. It was birthed from my personal training and nutrition career. One day my boss of many years, Roger Semsch, said, "Debbie how will you work 70 hours a week when your 60?" I said, "I will!" He said, "It's great that you are an amazing trainer but it would be even better if you trained others to be amazing?" So I did and we have Integrity. I've worked out of other gyms under the Integrity name hiring and managing trainers for almost 10 years now. We opened our own location in Winghaven in 2015. We also have a location in Clayton. Owning your own business is a humbling experience. My pay didn't get cut in half it got cut out! I learned to live on next to nothing, when prior to my hobby was buying handbags and new cars. :) Just kidding. I've always been humble but liked nice things. What was birthed through this was the clear and defined understanding that I truly serve my passion with what I do for a living. I serve God with this business and so does my amazing team. Each trainer cares for the client exactly the way I would, if not even better. Each trainer has his or her own specialty. They are truly amazing people. God gave me them. Without them Integrity would just be a name. Now it's a ministry to help people mind, body and spirit.

I've learned to live in lack and also with plenty. The one thing I could never live without is my relationship with Jesus Christ. He saved my life and healed my body. 20 years ago I saw a commercial on t.v. about Jesus, by my now pastor Jeff Perry at St. Louis Family Church. He had planted a seed in me that showed me I had hope. I was hopeless. I felt death was near and the doctors couldn't convince me otherwise. His salvation is why I am who I am today. Do you know Him? If not, ask Him into your heart. He will change your life forever.

Thank you Lord for the life you've given me.
Stay hungry for souls. My hope is in You, Lord.

Debbie Fottrell

www.integritytraininggroup.com

"the act of getting strong doesn't start in the gym. it starts in your head."

– unknown

Motivation

Bill & Barb's
Baked Green Beans

6 bags of Steam-in-Bag Green Beans
7 tbsp Olive Oil
1 tsp Sea Salt
1/2 tsp Pepper

Microwave all 6 bags per directions. Foil line a sheet cake pan. Spread green beans and combine with olive oil, salt and pepper. Bake at 350° for 30-45 minutes per desired doneness. Makes enough for the week.

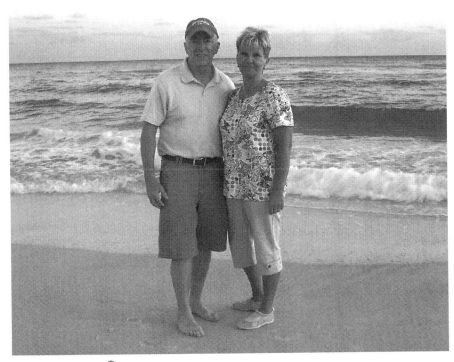

Train to Live · Food is Fuel

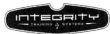

"i'm thankful for my struggle because without it i wouldn't have stumbled across my strength."

– unknown

Motivation

Bill & Barb's
Mashed Sweet Potatoes

6 medium Sweet Potatoes
1 tbsp Agave Nectar
1 tbsp Unsweetened Almond Milk
Stevia & Cinnamon to taste

Preheat oven to 400°. Wash sweet potatoes and lay on a cookie sheet. Bake for 90 minutes. Remove from oven and let cool. Peel off the skin and mash the sweet potatoes in a bowl. Add agave nectar, almond milk, and more cinnamon & stevia to taste. Blend with a hand mixer until smooth.

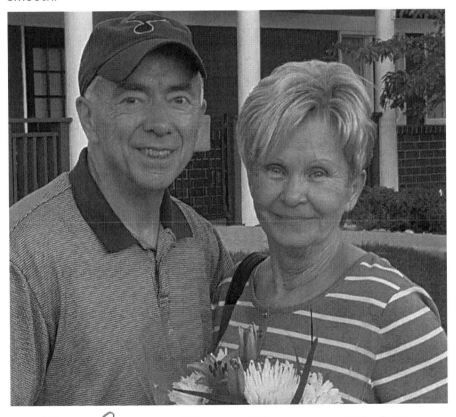

Train to Live · Food is Fuel
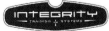

"we are what we repeatedly do. excellence then is not an act but a habit."

- Aristotle

Motivation

Bill & Barb's
Shredded BBQ Chicken

10-12 Boneless, Skinless Chicken Breasts
2 jars Bone Sucking Sauce (hot or mild)
Large crock pot

Rinse and place chicken breast in large crock pot. Pour entire jar of Bone Sucking BBQ sauce over chicken evenly. Cook on low for 10-12 hours. Drain chicken well. Place in a 13"x9" pan. Use two forks and shred the chicken. Pour the 2nd jar of Bone Sucking sauce over the chicken and stir well. Serve with baked green beans and baked sweet potatoes.

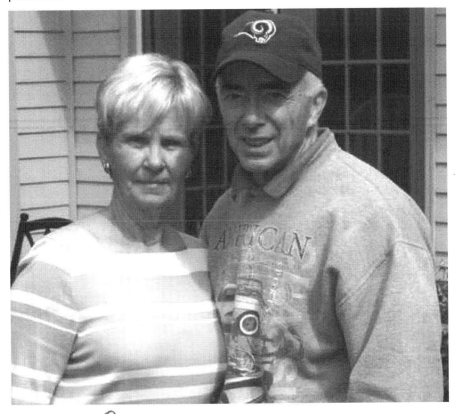

Train to Live · Food is Fuel

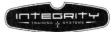

"the difference between the impossible and the possible lies in a person's determination."

- Tommy Lasorda

Motivation

Courtney's
Buffalo Turkey Meatballs
Courntey Stretar, Integrity Training Systems Personal Trainer

1 lb Ground Turkey
1 Egg
1/3 cup Almond Flour
2 tbsp of Primal Kitchen Mayonnaise
1/4 cup Frank's Hot Sauce
1/2 tsp of Salt and Pepper

Preheat oven to 400°. Combine all ingredients and mix well.
Using a small spoon or cookie scoop, dish out the turkey and roll into
balls. Place meat balls on cookie sheet. Bake for 20 minutes, flipping
halfway.
Serve with baked broccoli or zucchini noodles.

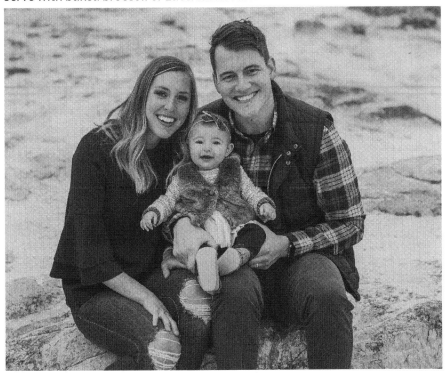

Train to Live . Food is Fuel

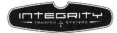

"if you want something you've never had, you must be willing to do something you've never done."

— Thomas Jefferson

Motivation

Debbie's

House Seasoning
Debbie Portell, Owner of Integrity Training Systems,
Personal Trainer & Nutrition Coach

1/2 cup Celtic Mineralized Sea Salt
1/4 cup Pepper
1/4 cup Garlic Powder
1 tbsp Onion Powder
1/4 tsp Cayenne Pepper

Combine all ingredients into a protein shaker, shake vigorously. Using a plastic funnel, pour mixture into a large, empty salt or pepper shaker. Add to your favorite dishes!

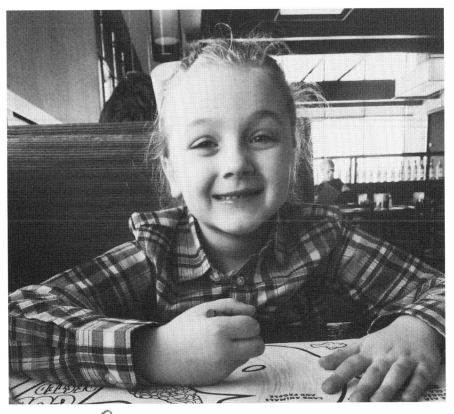

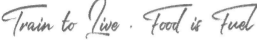

Train to Live . Food is Fuel

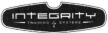

"fat lasts longer than flavor."

- unknown

Motivation

Dr. Ian's
Balsamic Glazed Chicken & Roasted Veggie Bowl

Dr. Ian McDonald, Chapel McMurtrie Bartlett Chiropractic

16 oz Chicken Breast cut into 1/4" chunks
16 oz Brussels Sprouts, trimmed, large sprouts halves or quartered
16 oz Sweet Potatoes (about 1 large), cut into 1/2 inch cubes
2 tbsp Olive Oil
1/2 cup Balsamic Vinegar (*optional*)
1/4 cup Almond or Brazil Nuts, toasted and coarsely chopped
1/2 cup Brown Rice (*optional*)
2 oz Low-Fat Goat Cheese (*optional*)

Preheat oven to 400°F. Combine brussels sprouts and sweet potatoes in a large bowl with olive oil and black pepper; toss to coat. Transfer to a large, rimmed baking sheet. Roast 30–35 minutes, stirring in the cut chicken and with 8–10 minutes remaining. Cook rice as noted on box. *Optional step:* While vegetables roast, add balsamic vinegar to a small saucepan and simmer over medium heat until reduced by at least half, about 11–13 minutes. Remove from heat and set aside. Once chicken is warmed through, remove pan from the oven and transfer contents to a large serving bowl. Add balsamic vinegar and chopped hazelnuts and gently toss to coat. Divide into individual serving bowls and top each with rice and 1/2 ounce goat cheese crumbles, if desired. Serve warm.

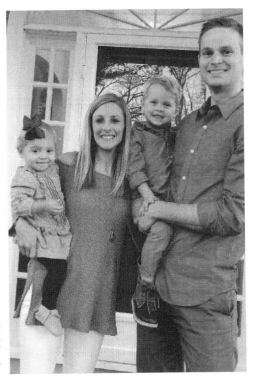

Train to Live . Food is Fuel

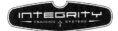

"to give anything less than your best is to sacrifice the gift."

- Steve Prefontaine

Motivation

Dover's
Dandy Jerky
Dr. Ava Frick, Pet Rehab & Pain Clinic

The best snack for our pooch friends, especially those who are a bit of a poofy pooch, is home-made dehydrated meat. No preservatives or artificial flavorings. No flour. And the best is, no calorie counting required when given in small amounts. (Cats like this snack too!)
Time to clean last year's venison out of the freezer to make space for the new deer trophy.

Meat (*Venison, Beef, Bison Roast*) or Organs (*Lung, Liver, Spleen, Kidney*)
Olive Oil, Grape Seed Oil or Walnut Oil
Sea Salt (gray or pink)

Defrost until firm but not solid so that it can easily be sliced thin. Lightly spread a cookie sheet with oil of your choice (to prevent the meat from sticking). Place the thin sliced meat onto the cookie sheet, covering it (*Dover wanted those last 2 words added*) Sprinkle moderately with sea salt. Put into oven and set on low temperature of 150° to dehydrate the meat or organ. Let cook for several hours to overnight until is crispy and will break when bent. Or use that dehydrator you have and follow directions. Break up into little, smaller than bite size pieces. (*Dover wanted me to say, "Generous, larger than bite size pieces." But I didn't. Don't let him know I gypped on the size of the jerky pieces. Shhh!*)
Cool until no heat or moisture remains in the meat or organ. Store in a glass container with sealed lid. If you have thoroughly dehydrated it the jerky will keep for months. Get what you need for the day and take with you where ever you and your pooch go. Keep those fitness exercise lessons coming!

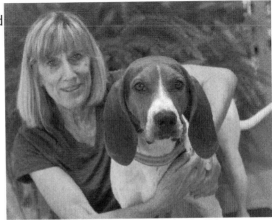

Train to Live . Food is Fuel

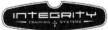

"the secret of change is to focus all of your energy, not on fighting the old, but on building the new."

- Socrates

Motivation

Forrest's

Arugula Pesto
Forrest Boston, Integrity Training Systems Personal Trainer

(This pesto is great on everything: stirred into scrambled eggs, spread on sandwiches, mixed with roasted potatoes and stirred into pasta.)

2 Cloves of Garlic, Peeled
6 cups Arugula
1 cup Fresh Basil
1 cup Toasted Walnuts
1/2 cup Extra-Virgin Olive Oil
3 tbsp Grated Parmesan Cheese
2 tbsp Lemon Juice

In a food processor process garlic until chopped. Add arugula and basil; process until minced. Add walnuts, olive oil, cheese, lemon juice, 1/2 tsp salt, and 1/4 tsp black pepper. Process until smooth and creamy. Makes 1 2/3 cups. *Make-ahead tip:* Refrigerate in an airtight container up to 5 days.
Per 1 Tbsp. 71 cal, 7 g fat, 33 mg sodium, 1 g carb, 1 g protein

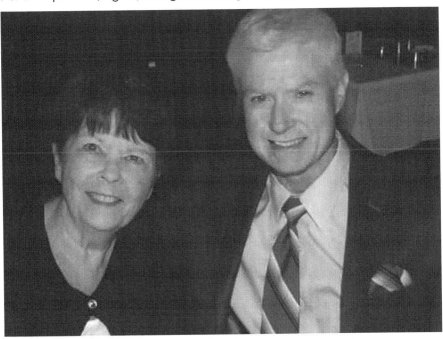

Train to Live · Food is Fuel

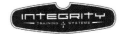

"impossible is just an opinion."

- Paulo Coelho

Forrest's Chicken-Zucchini Meatballs

Forrest Boston, Integrity Training Systems Personal Trainer

1 cup Finely Shredded Zucchini
1 lb Ground Chicken
1 Egg, Lightly Beaten
1/2 cup Gluten-Free Panko
1/2 cup Grated Parmesan Cheese
2 Cloves of Garlic, Minced
1 tbsp Chopped Fresh Parsley
2 tsp Dried Basil, Crushed
1/4 tsp Crushed Red Pepper

Preheat oven to 350 °. Line a 15" x 10" baking pan with foil; coat with nonstick cooking spray. Line a colander with paper towels; add zucchini. Sprinkle 1/8 tsp salt over zucchini. Let stand 20 minutes, pressing occasionally to remove moisture. In a large bowl combine zucchini, chicken, egg, panko, cheese, garlic, parsley, basil, crushed red pepper, and 1/8 tsp salt. Shape rounded tablespoons of mixture into 20 meatballs; place in prepared pan. Bake 25 minutes or until cooked through (165°). *Makes 20. Make-ahead tip: Refrigerate in an airtight container up to 5 days or freeze up to 3 months.*
Per Meatball 103 cal, 5 g fat, 61 mg chol, 175 mg sodium, 3 g carb, 10 g protein

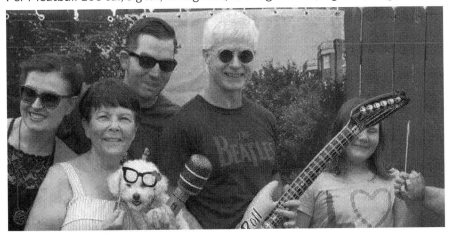

Train to Live . Food is Fuel

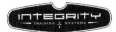

" don't let your weekend

become your weak end."

– unknown

Motivation

Julie's

Chili Dogs

Julie Marling, Integrity Training Systems Personal Trainer

1 Package of Applegate Hot Dogs
3 Sweet Potatoes
Your favorite chili recipe
Cheese for topping

Heat oven 425°. Bake potatoes for 45 minutes until tender. Prepare the hot dogs and chili. Halve the potatoes and scoop out some flesh.
Turn oven to broil and put a hot dog and chili inside each sweet potato. Top with cheese. Place in oven until the cheese is melted

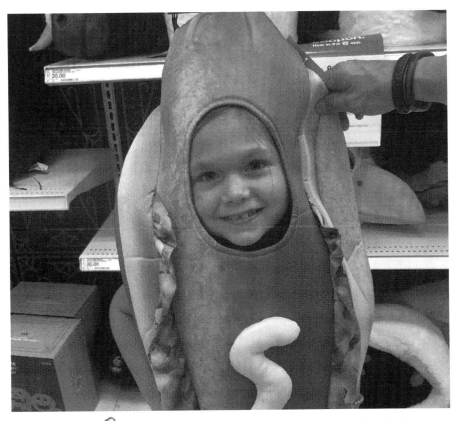

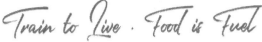

Train to Live · Food is Fuel

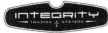

"a goal without a plan is just a wish."

– Antoine de Saint-Exupéry

Motivation

Julie's Granola Bars

Julie Marling, Integrity Training Systems Personal Trainer

1 ³/₄ cup of Quick-Cooking Oats
2/3 cup of Enjoy Life Dark Chocolate Chips
1 tsp of Cinnamon
Salt to taste
1 cup of Natural Peanut Butter
1/2 cup of Honey
2 tsp of Alcohol-Free Vanilla Extract

Grease 8" baker pan or granola bar snack maker. Mix oats, chips, cinnamon and salt. In another bowl mix the remaining ingredients. Tip warm the mixture in the microwave so it will mix better with the dry ingredients. Just let it cool so it doesn't melt your chocolate chips. Mix the wet and dry ingredients. Make sure there is no dry oats left in the bowl. Transfer the mixture to your pan of choice and use a spoon to firmly press into the pan. Cover and refrigerate for 1 hour. Use a sharp knife and slice into bars.

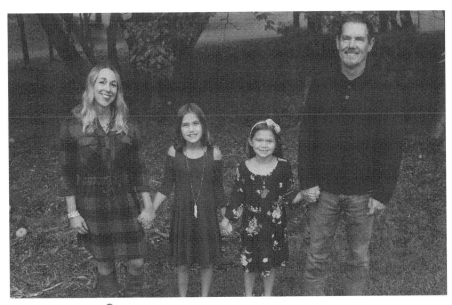

Train to Live . Food is Fuel

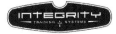

"every 365 days, your skin replaces itself. your liver, about a month. your body makes these new cells from the food you eat. what you eat literally becomes you. you have a choice in what you're made of. eat wisely."

— unknown

Motivation

Julie's

Green Juice
Julie Marling, Integrity Training Systems Personal Trainer

4-5 Green Apples
1 Lemon
4 Stalks of Celery
1 Cucumber
Handful of Spinach and Kale

Place all the ingredients into a juicer. Once it is complete I pour into jars. I fill the jar about 3/4 full then top the rest with water. I place them in the freezer. Each day my girls drink a cup of green juice. 1 jar is enough for 2-4 glasses of juice. This recipe yields 6-8 jars of green juice.

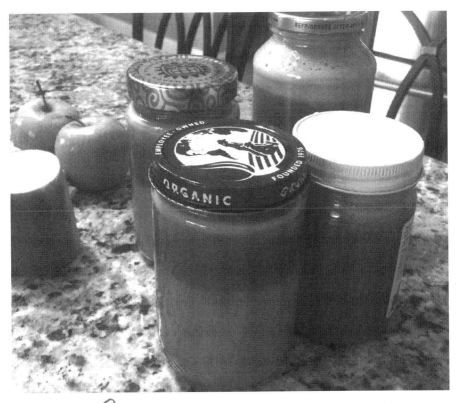

Train to Live . Food is Fuel

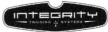

"you messed up your diet & you didn't exercise today-so what? you didn't ruin anything. get back on track tomorrow. if you have one flat tire, do you slash the other three? of course not."

- Jillian Michaels

Motivation

Julie's Protein Lasagna

Julie Marling, Integrity Training Systems Personal Trainer
- adapted from Maria Emmerich

1 lb of Grass-Fed Beef
1/4 Diced Onion
1 Clove of Garlic
2 cups of Raos Marinara Sauce or any low sugar sauce
1 lb of Shaved Turkey Breast (I have the deli cut it a little thicker than
    regular sandwich meat)
2 cups of Cottage Cheese
2 cups of Mozzarella Cheese
1/4 cup of Parmesan Cheese

Brown the hamburger, onion and garlic. Then add marinara sauce. Mix all your cheeses in a separate bowl. Grease your slow cooker. Spread layer of meat sauce on bottom of slow cooker. Then add a scoop of cheese mix. Last, add a layer of noodles (turkey meat) across the cheese mixture. Repeat pattern. The last layer should be the cheese mixture. Top with Parmesan cheese. Cook on low for 3-4 hours. Let it rest for 1 hour before serving.

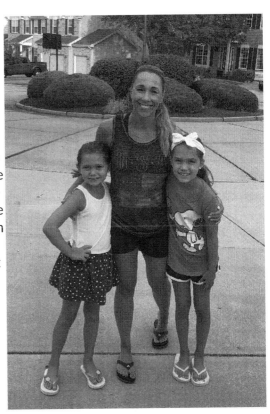

Train to Live · Food is Fuel

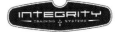

"making excuses burns zero
calories per hour."

– unknown

Motivation

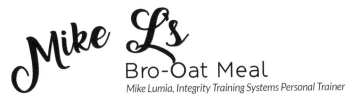

Mike L's
Bro-Oat Meal
Mike Lumia, Integrity Training Systems Personal Trainer

1/2-1 cup Old-Fashion Oats
1-1 $^{1/2}$ scoops of your favorite Protein Powder
    (I use Jay Rob Chocolate Egg White Protein)
Unsweetened Cocoa
1-2 tbsp of your favorite Natural Nut Butter (*no-sugar added*)
Riced Cauliflower (*optional lower carb option*)

Cook oats as suggested, then let cool in fridge. After cooled add protein, cocoa and nut butter. Mix and put in the freezer until it's consistently you like. You also wait to add nut butter on top. *If you're on a lower carb diet, use less oats & add frozen plain riced cauliflower as a filler.*

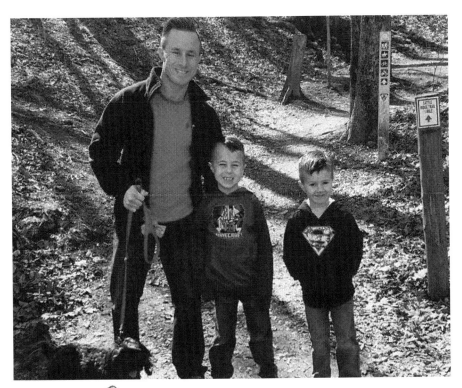

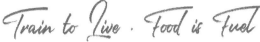

Train to Live . Food is Fuel

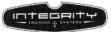

"create healthy habits, not restrictions."

– unknown

Motivation

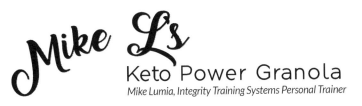

Mike L's
Keto Power Granola
Mike Lumia, Integrity Training Systems Personal Trainer

1 ¹/² cups Almonds
1 ¹/² cups Pecans
1 cup Almond Flour
1/4 cup Sunflower Seeds
1/3 cup Swerve Granular Sweetener
1/3 cup Vanilla Whey Protein Powder
1/3 cup Natural Peanut Butter
1/4 cup Grass-Fed Butter
1/4 cup Water

Preheat oven to 300° and line a large rimmed baking sheet with parchment paper. In a food processor, process almonds and pecans until they resemble coarse crumbs with some larger pieces. Transfer to a large bowl and stir in, sunflower seeds, sweetener, and vanilla protein powder. In a microwave safe bowl, melt the peanut butter and butter together. Pour melted peanut butter mixture over nut mixture and stir well, tossing lightly. Stir in water. Mixture will clump together. Spread mixture evenly on prepared baking sheet and bake 30 minutes, stirring halfway through. Remove and let cool completely.

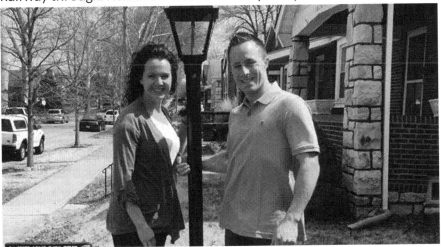

Train to Live . Food is Fuel

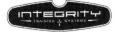

"fitness isn't a seasonal hobby, it's a lifestyle."

– unknown

Motivation

Sheila's
Avocado Bacon & Eggs
Sheila Stender, Integrity Training Systems Personal Trainer

1 medium Avocado
2 Eggs
1 strip of Cooked Bacon, Crumbled (Uncured Bacon with No-Sugar Added)
1 tbsp Shredded Cheese
Sea salt

Preheat the oven to 425°. Cut the avocado in half and remove the pit. Scoop out the center of each half of the avocado, big enough to accommodate the eggs. Place in a muffin pan to stabilize the avocado while cooking. Put 1 egg in each half of the avocado. Sprinkle the top with cheese, crumbled bacon and a dash of sea salt. Cook 14 to 16 minutes. Serve warm.

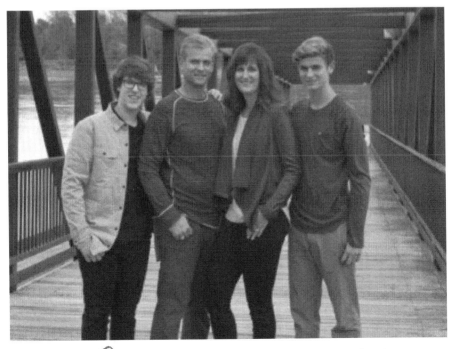

Train to Live · Food is Fuel

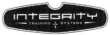

"there are 7 days in a workweek and someday isn't one of them."

– unknown

Motivation

Sheila's

Pizza Stuffed Chicken Breast
Sheila Stender, Integrity Training Systems Personal Trainer

4 Chicken Breasts
1 cup of Marinara Sauce (no-sugar added)
1 cup of Shredded Mozzarella Cheese
1 tbsp Italian Seasonings
Choice of pizza toppings (peppers, onions, mushrooms, tomatoes, broccoli)

Slice the chicken breasts in the middle and stuff with pizza toppings and shredded cheese. Baste the top of the chicken with olive oil and drizzle marinara sauce over the breasts, enough to cover the chicken. Sprinkle with Italian seasonings. Bake at 350° for 25 minutes or until the chicken is cooked through.

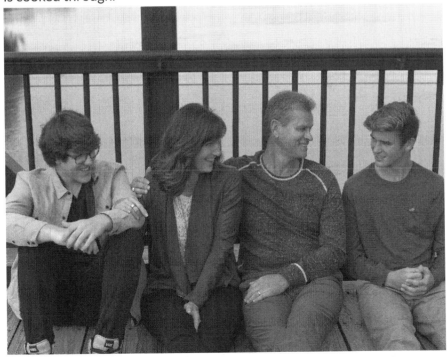

Train to Live · Food is Fuel

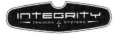

it does not matter how slowly you go as long as you do not stop.

– Confucius

Motivation

Sophie's
After Dinner Snack

1 whole Peach, cubed
1/2 tsp Cinnamon
1/2 tsp Alcohol-Free Vanilla
1 dash Now Foods Pure Stevia
2 tsp Avocado Oil
1 Gluten-Free Graham Cracker, crumbled

Sauté the peach in the avocado oil. Add all remaining ingredients except the graham cracker. Combine and cook down the peach until soft but still solid. Place graham cracker in a Ziploc bag and crumble well. Add to the top of the peach. Enjoy!

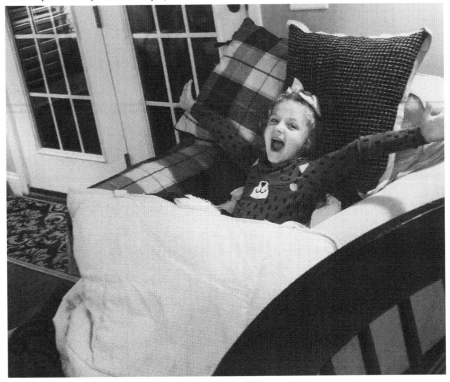

Train to Live . Food is Fuel

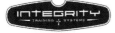

"it's going to be a journey. it's not a sprint to get in shape."

- Kerri Walsh Jenning

Motivation

$\mathcal{S}$ophie's
After School Snack

2 Hard Boiled Eggs
1 tbsp Primal Avocado Mayo
dash of Now Foods Pure Stevia
dash of Salt and Pepper

Slice eggs in half. Set aside yolks in a bowl. Combine remaining ingredients to egg yolk. Fill in the egg white to make a deviled egg. Great snack full of protein and quality fat!

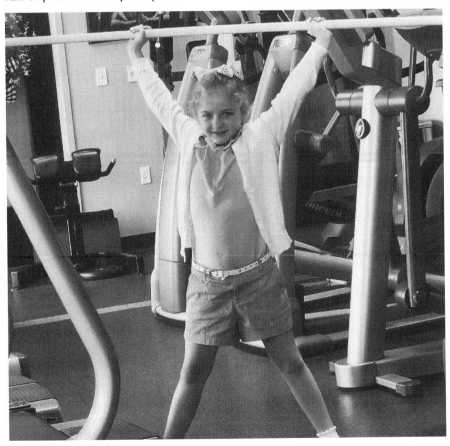

Train to Live . Food is Fuel

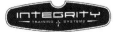

"life has no limitations,
except the ones you make."

- Les Brown

Motivation

Sophie's Apple Cinnamon Protein Muffins

2 scoops Vanilla Egg White Protein Powder
1/2 scoop Cinnamon Apple Ancient Nutrition Collagen Protein Powder
2 tbsp Unsweetened Vanilla Coconut Milk
1/2 cup Almond Butter
1 heaping cup Unsweetened Cinnamon Applesauce
1 tsp Alcohol-Free Vanilla
1 tsp Cinnamon
1 tsp Aluminum-Free Baking Powder
1/2 cup Golden Raisins

Mix all ingredients, setting raisins aside. Once mixed well, fold raisins in. Spray pan completely with soy-free coconut oil spray. Cook at 350° for 20 to 25 minutes or until a knife comes clean from testing.

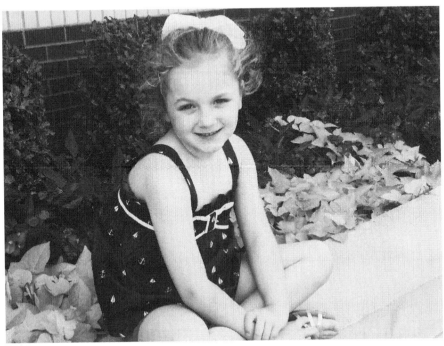

Train to Live · Food is Fuel

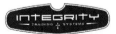

"no matter how many mistakes you make or how slow you progress, you are still way ahead of everyone who isn't trying."

– Tony Robbins

Motivation

Sophie's
Apple Pie Protein Muffins

1/2 cup So Delicious Unsweetened Vanilla Coconut Milk Yogurt
1/2 cup Cinnamon Unsweetened Applesauce
2 cups Gluten-Free Oats
1 scoop Ancient Nutrition Apple Cinnamon Bone Broth Protein Powder
1 scoop Vanilla Egg White or Collagen Powder
1/3 cup Pure Maple Syrup
2 Eggs
1 tsp Alcohol-Free Vanilla
1 tsp Cinnamon
1 tsp Baking Powder
1/4 tsp Sea Salt
1 cup Apple, peeled and chopped

A lower sugar option would be to replace maple syrup with Stevia.

Blend all ingredients, leaving apple until last. Fold in Apple. Pour into muffin tins or mini loaf pans. Cook at 350° for 30 minutes.

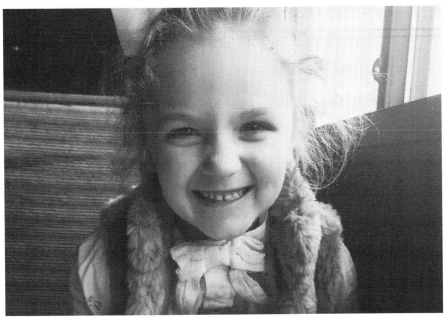

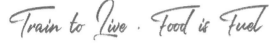

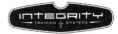

"success is never on discount! greatness is never on sale! greatness is never half off! it's all or nothing! it's all day, every day! greatness is never on discount!"

- Eric Thomas

Motivation

Sophie's Bacon Wrapped Asparagus

1 bundle of Thick Asparagus Spears, *cut at where bottom rubber band is*
8 strips of Bacon, Pederson's Uncured, No-Sugar Added
Avocado Oil
Onion Powder, *sprinkle across the spears*
Celtic Sea Salt, to taste
Pepper, to taste
Unbleached Parchment Paper

Preheat oven to 375°. Place parchment paper inside sheet cake pan,

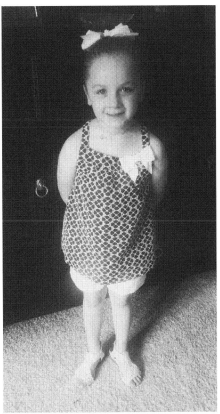

lay asparagus on top of that. Drizzle avocado oil over the top of the asparagus. Take a strip of bacon and wrap around the asparagus, avoid overlapping. Continue to wrap each spear until gone. Set each bundle on top of wire cooling rack and place that inside of sheet cake pan. Put extra spears without bacon on the open space of the rack. Every 5-8 minutes flip the bundle, cook the bundles for 25-30 minutes, more if you like the bacon crispier. Check plain asparagus spears periodically until to the doneness you prefer. Enjoy!

Train to Live . Food is Fuel

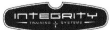

"you can either suffer the pain of discipline or the pain of regret."

- Jim Rohn

Motivation

Sophie's
Bacon Wrapped Hot dogs

8 Hot Dogs Uncured, No-Sugar Added
8 strips of Bacon Uncured, No-Sugar Added

Cut a strip through each hot dog to butterfly them. You don't want to cut them in half, just right before. Wrap each hot dog with bacon. Place a cooling rack inside a sheet cake pan. I put parchment paper down on the sheet cake pan to lessen the clean up. Spread the hot dogs out evenly on the cooling rack. Cook on 350° for 15 minutes on one side, flip them and 15 minutes on the other side.

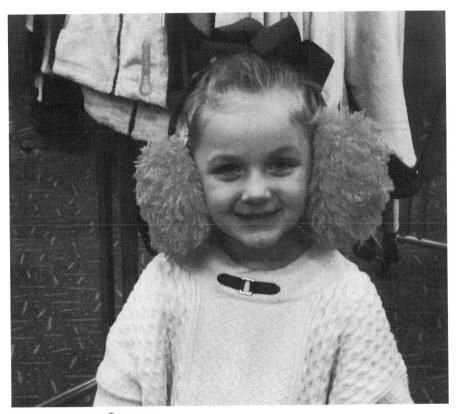

Train to Live . Food is Fuel

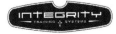

"if it doesn't challenge you it doesn't change you!"

- Fred Devito

Motivation

Sophie's Banana Nut Protein Muffins

2 scoops Vanilla Egg White Protein Powder
1 tsp Aluminum-Free Baking Powder
1/2 cup Almond Flour
1/2 cup Raw Almond or Cashew Butter
2 Mashed Ripe Bananas
1 tsp Alcohol-Free Vanilla
2 tbsp Unsweetened Vanilla Coconut Milk
1 tsp Cinnamon
1/4 tsp Sea Salt
1 tbsp Pure Maple Syrup
1/2 cup Chopped Walnuts or Pecans

Blend all ingredients, leaving nuts aside. Spray muffin pan well with soy-free coconut oil cooking spray. Fold in nuts. Distribute batter evenly. Bake at 350° for 15 minutes.

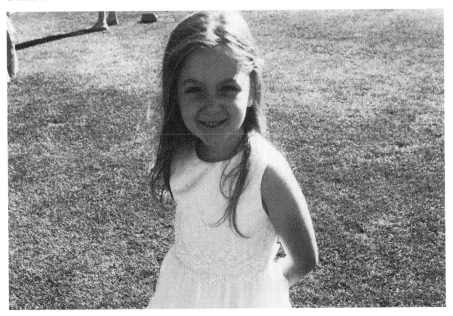

Train to Live . Food is Fuel

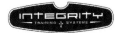

"the voice in your head
that says you can't do this
is a liar."

– unknown

Motivation

Sophie's Banana Peanut Butter Sandwich

1 piece Udis Cinnamon Raisin Bread
1/2 tbsp Natural Peanut Butter
4 thin slices of Banana
1 dash of Now Foods Pure Stevia
1 dash of Cinnamon

Toast the bread. Spread the peanut butter. Place banana slices in top.
Mix cinnamon and stevia together and drizzle over the top. Serve with
coconut milk blended with vanilla egg white protein powder and
cinnamon.

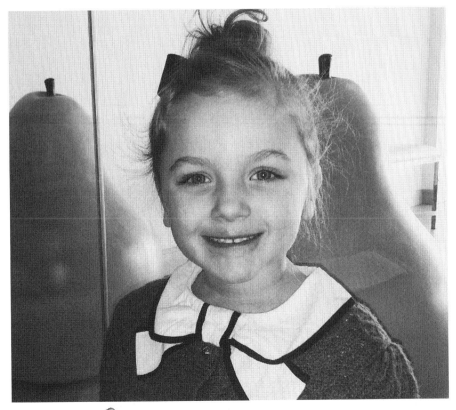

Train to live . Food is Fuel

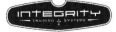

"every day is another chance to get stronger, to eat better, to live healthier, and to be the best version of you."

- unknown

Motivation

Sophie's
Bedtime Snack

Serve warm and pour the cold yogurt over the top

idea

1 Apple
1 tsp Cinnamon
1 tsp Alcohol-Free Vanilla
1/2 tbsp Avocado Oil
1/2 scoop Cinnamon-Apple Ancient Nutrition Bone Broth
       Protein Powder
1/2 cup Unsweetened Vanilla So Delicious Coconut Milk Yogurt
1 dash Now Foods Pure Stevia Powder
Walnuts or Pecans (*optional*)

Chop the apple and sauté in avocado oil until soft. Add half of the vanilla and cinnamon to the apples. Set aside. Thoroughly blend the ingredients in a blender or food processor. Pour on top of the apple. Top with chopped pecans or walnuts (optional), they can even be toasted with the apple.

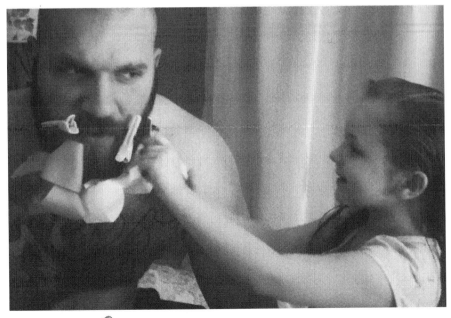

Train to Live · Food is Fuel

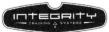

"the same voice that says 'give up' can also be trained to say 'keep going'."

– unknown

Motivation

Sophie's
Berry Power Smoothie
-with electrolytes

1 cup Mixed Berries, including Cherries
1 Cherry or Blackberry Hint Water
2 dashes of Now Foods Pure Stevia Powder
1 scoop Vital Proteins Collagen Peptides Unflavored
1 tbsp Barlean's Blueberry Pomegranate Flax Oil
1 packet of Cherry or Berry Ultima Electrolyte Powder

Combine all ingredients into a blender at one time. Fruit can be fresh or frozen. Blend well. This is a great source of fuel prior to a sporting event. An excellent source of protein, fat, carbs and electrolytes.

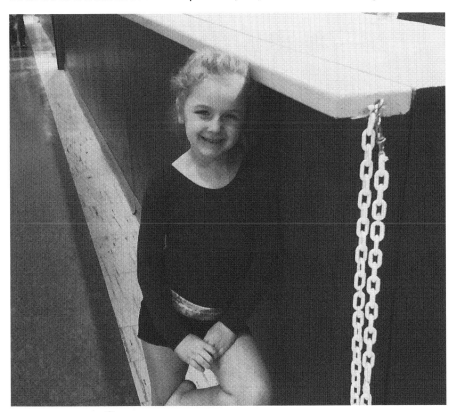

Train to Live . Food is Fuel

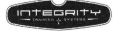

"motivation is what gets you started. habit is what keeps you going."

- Jim Ryin

Motivation

Sophie's
BLT Wrap

2 strips Uncured No-Sugar Added Turkey Bacon
2 slices of Tomato
1/2 Hard Boiled Egg, sliced
2 large Leaves of Lettuce
Pinch of Sea Salt
1/2 tbsp Chipotle Primal Avocado Mayo

Instead of using bread we double up the lettuce. We spread the mayo on the lettuce. We wrap the egg, bacon and tomato together and pinch the salt over the eggs and tomato.

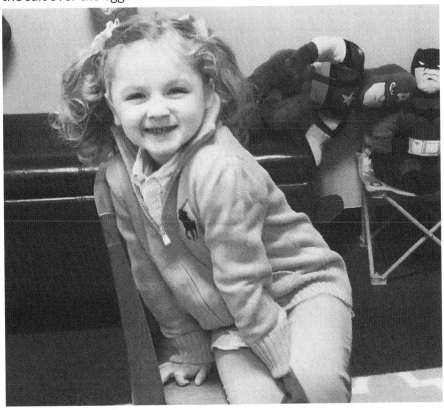

Train to Live . Food is Fuel

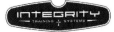

"exercise should be regarded
as a tribute to the heart."

- Gene Tunney

Sophie's
Blueberry Power Yogurt

1 cup Unsweetened Vanilla So Delicious Coconut Milk Yogurt
1/2 cup Blueberries
1/2 scoop Vanilla Jay Rob Egg White Protein Powder
1 tbsp Blueberry Pomegranate Barlean's Flax Seed Oil
1 dash of Now Foods Pure Stevia Powder

Blend all ingredients in your blender. I like to use frozen berries that are thawed that create a juice. These are also great frozen in Popsicle molds.

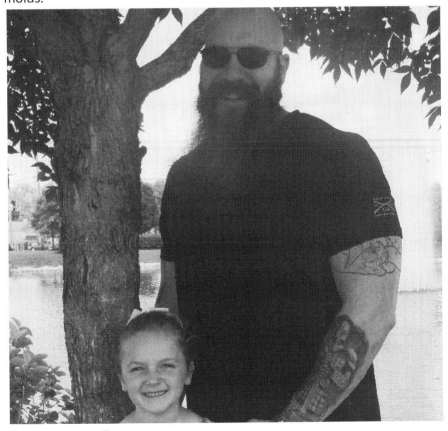

Train to Live . Food is Fuel

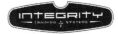

"everybody has a dream, but not everybody has a grind."

- Eric Thomas

Motivation

Sophie's
Blueberry Vanilla Protein Muffins

2 ¼ cup Gluten-Free Oats
1 Mashed Banana
1/4 cup Pure Maple Syrup
1/2 tsp Alcohol-Free Vanilla
1 ½ scoops Vanilla Egg White or Collagen Powder
1/3 cup Natural Peanut or Cashew Butter
1 Egg
1/4 cup Unsweetened Applesauce
1 tsp Aluminum-Free Baking Powder
1/4 tsp Sea Salt
1 cup Unsweetened Vanilla Coconut Milk
1 cup Blueberries

Blend all ingredients, leaving nuts aside. Spray muffin pan well with soy-free coconut oil cooking spray. Fold in nuts. Distribute batter evenly. Bake at 350° for 15 minutes.

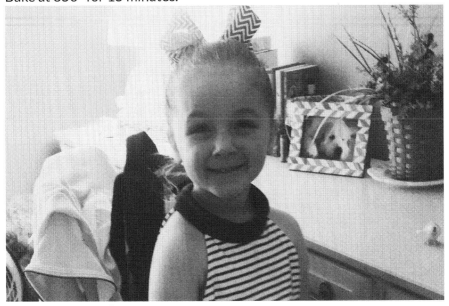

Train to Live . Food is Fuel

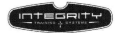

"the only bad workout is
the one that didn't

happen."

- unknown

Motivation

Sophie's
Buffalo Chicken Sandwich

2 Chicken Cutlets
1 cup Almond Flour
1 tbsp Garlic Powder
1/2 tsp Paprika
1/4 tsp Salt
1/4 tsp Pepper
2 large Eggs
1/2 cup Frank's Hot Sauce
1/4 cup Avocado Oil
Pinch Now Foods Pure Stevia
1/2 tbsp Lemon Juice
Ziploc bag

Preheat oven to 350°. Combine dry ingredients. Add them to a large Ziploc bag. Dredge breasts into the eggs. Drop breast into bag and shake until well coated. Sear for 5 mins on each side in a grill pan add grill pan to preheated oven and cook for 10-15 minutes. Combine remaining ingredients and pour on top of chicken. Cook for 5 more minutes. Serve on top of lettuce with avocado mayo. I like to add grilled onions on top as well.

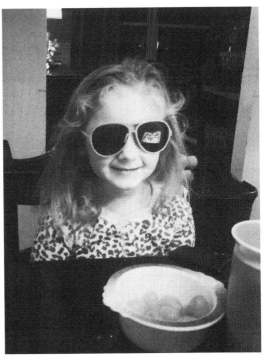

Train to Live . Food is Fuel

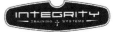

"a one hour workout is

4% of your day.

No excuses!"

– unknown

Motivation

Sophie's
Carrot Cake Protein Muffins

1/2 cup Unsweetened Vanilla So Delicious Coconut Milk Yogurt
3/4 cup of Pineapple Puree (blend 1 1/2 cups of pineapple)
1/2 cup Shredded Carrots
2 scoops Vanilla Egg White or Collagen Powder
2 Eggs
1 tsp Alcohol-Free Vanilla
1 tsp Cinnamon
1 tsp Aluminum-Free Baking Powder
1/2 tsp Salt

Blend all ingredients until combined well. Pour into muffin cups. Cook at 350° for 30 minutes.

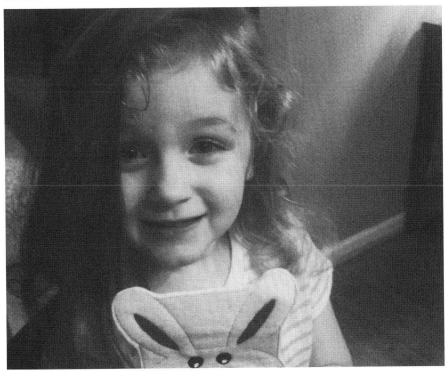

Train to Live . Food is Fuel

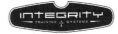

"'i don't have time' is the grown-up version of 'the dog ate my homework'."

– unknown

Motivation

Sophie's
Cauliflower Mexican Rice

1 bag of Frozen Green Giant Riced Cauliflower
2 tbsp Avocado Oil
1/2 cup No-Sugar Salsa
1/2 cup Diced Onion
1 cup Green, Red and Yellow Peppers, combined
1/2 can Chopped, Diced Tomatoes
1/2 cup No-Sugar Guacamole

Microwave cauliflower per directions on bag. Sauté all ingredients except salsa for 15 to 20 minutes or until desired doneness, stirring often. Add in the salsa, stir in well. Top with guacamole.

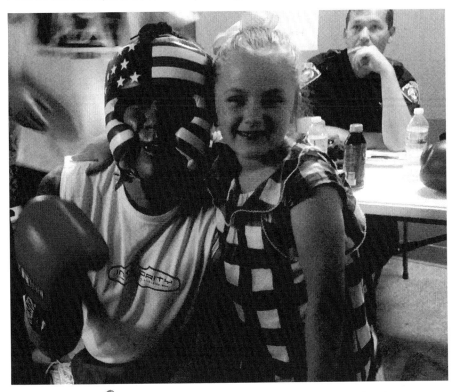

Train to Live · Food is Fuel

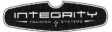

"one workout at a time.

one day at a time.

one meal at a time."

- Chalene Johnson

Motivation

Sophie's
Cherry Protein Popsicle

1 cup Pitted Cherries or thawed, frozen
1 Cherry Hint Water
2 pinches of Now Foods Pure Stevia Powder
1 scoop Vital Proteins Collagen Peptides Unflavored

Blend all ingredients well until liquefied. Pour into Popsicle molds.
Freeze for 30 minutes. Enjoy!

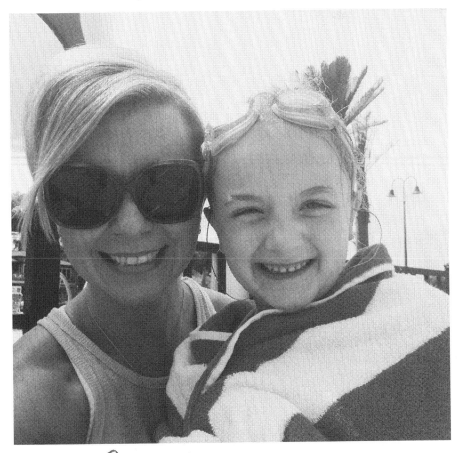

Train to Live . Food is Fuel

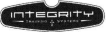

"you are capable of

great things."

– unknown

Motivation

Sophie's
Chicken Tenders

1 Package Bare Chicken Tenderloins
2 Egg Whites
2 $^{1/2}$ - 3 cups Bobs Red Mill Almond Flour
1 tbsp Celtic Sea Salt
1/2 tbsp Pepper
2 tbsp Parsley
1 tsp Paprika
1 tsp Garlic Granules
2 tsp Onion Powder
1 $^{1/2}$ tbsp Avocado Oil

Preheat oven to 350°. Coat the Bare Chicken Tenderloins in egg whites then immediately coat with the almond flour mixture. Place in griddle pan with heated avocado oil, cook each side to a crispy golden brown. Once cooked, put a sheet of parchment paper inside a sheet cake pan (for easy clean up), then place a metal wire cooking rack on top of that. Place cooked chicken on top of rack and place in the oven. Cook until chicken is cooked through, about an additional 8 minutes. Serve with a side of your favorite veggies.

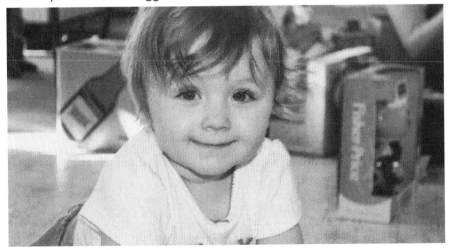

Train to Live . Food is Fuel

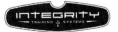

"strength doesn't come from what you can do. it comes from overcoming the things you once thought you couldn't."

- Ashley Greene

Motivation

Sophie's
Chili

1 Orange Pepper	1 tbsp Frank's Hot Sauce
1 Red Pepper	6 Stalks of Celery
2 Green Peppers	1/2 small can of Tomato Paste
1 Yellow Pepper	2 cans of Chopped Tomatoes
1 large Onion	1 dash Red Pepper Flakes
3 tbsp Chili Powder	1 dash Cayenne
2 tbsp Onion Powder	1 tbsp Garlic Powder
1 tbsp Sea Salt	2 tbsp Black Pepper
2 tbsp Stevia	1/4 cup Bone Sucking Sauce
2 large cans of Tomato Sauce	3 lbs Ground Turkey or Bison

Chop and sauté the veggies in olive oil, cook meat separately and drain. Add all ingredients together. Stir well, cook on medium for 30 minutes. Tastes great served over roasted spaghetti squash.

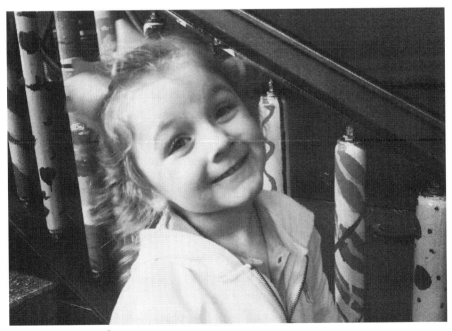

Train to Live . Food is Fuel

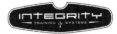

"your fitness is 100%
mental. your body won't
go where your mind doesn't
push it."

- unknown

Motivation

Sophie's
Chocolate Banana Protein Frozen Yogurt

2 cups Unsweetened Vanilla So Delicious Coconut Milk Yogurt
2 scoops Chocolate Egg White or Collagen Powder
2 dash Now Foods Pure Stevia Powder
1 whole Banana
2 tbsp Natural Peanut Butter

Blend all ingredients until well combined. Pour into Popsicle molds. Freeze for at least 30 minutes. Enjoy!

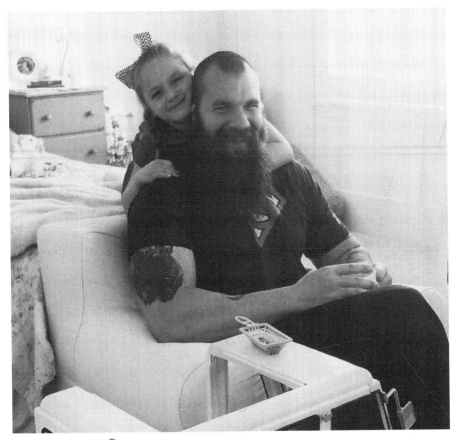

Train to Live . Food is Fuel

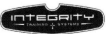

"our bodies are capable of anything. it's our minds we have to convince."

– unknown

Motivation

Sophie's Chocolate Brownie Protein Energy Balls

1/2 cup Almond Flour
1 scoop Chocolate Egg White Protein Powder
2 tbsp Cocoa Powder
2 tbsp Natural Peanut, Almond or Cashew Butter
2 tbsp Maple Syrup
2 tbsp Coconut Milk
2 tbsp Gluten-Free, Dairy-Free Mini Chocolate Chips
2 tbsp Unsweetened Golden Raisins

Blend all ingredients well. Fold chips and raisins in. Roll into tbsp size balls. Place on parchment paper. Keep stored in the refrigerator or freezer.

idea

A lower sugar option would be to replace maple syrup with Stevia.

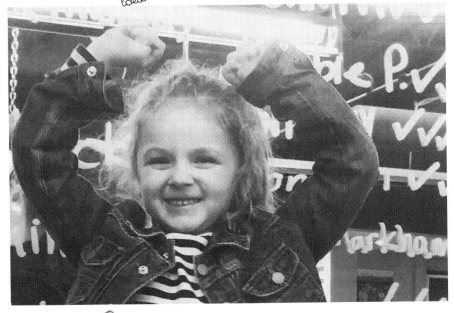

Train to Live . Food is Fuel

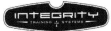

"commitment means staying loyal to what you said you were going to do long after the mood you said it in has left you."

- unknown

Motivation

Sophie's
Chocolate Chip Protein Muffins

2 scoops Vanilla Egg White or Collagen Powder
1 tsp Baking Powder
1/2 cup Almond Flour
1/2 cup Natural Peanut, Almond or Cashew Butter
1 cup Unsweetened Apple Sauce
1 tsp Alcohol-Free Vanilla
1 tbsp Pure Maple Syrup or Honey
1/2 cup Gluten-Free, Dairy-Free Chocolate Chips

Combine all ingredients and mix well. Fold chips in. Pour into muffin tins. Bake at 350° for 15 minutes.

idea
A lower sugar option would be to replace maple syrup with Stevia.

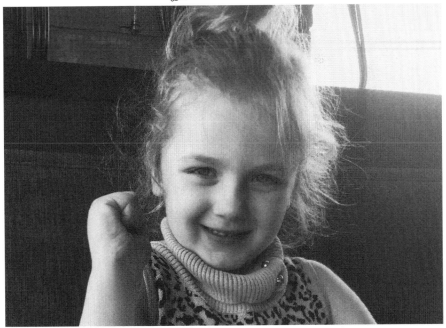

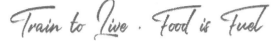
Train to Live · Food is Fuel

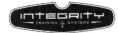

"it's never too late to
change your life."

- unknown

Motivation

Sophie's
Chocolate Covered Cherries

1 bag Frozen Cherries, thawed
1/2 cup Gluten and Dairy-Free Chocolate Chips
1 cup So Delicious Coconut Milk Whipped Cream

Warm cherries in a bowl for 1 minute with chocolate on top. Stir well and warm for another 15 to 30 seconds. Top with coconut whipped cream.

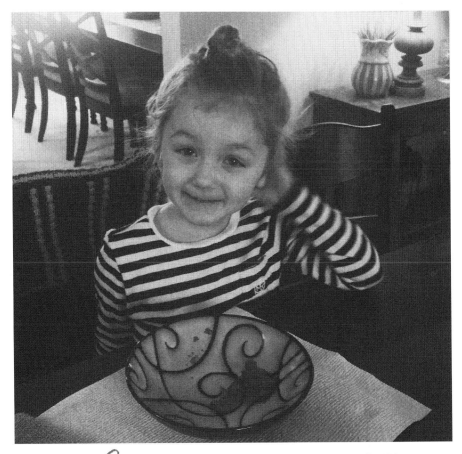

Train to Live . Food is Fuel

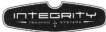

"health is not about the weight you lose, but the life you gain!"

- Dr. Josh Axe

Motivation

Sophie's
Chocolate Ice Cream

2 Frozen Bananas
1/2 cup Almond or Coconut Milk
2 scoops Jay Robb's Chocolate Protein Powder
1/2 tbsp Cocoa Powder
Strawberries and Blueberries (*optional*)

Put frozen chopped up bananas in blender/Ninja & blend, then add other ingredients! Put in a freezable container & freeze until more solid, Enjoy! Sophie likes to add the strawberries and blueberries on top of her ice cream.Glad containers work for freezing it in! *Note: if all of it doesn't get eaten, put back in freezer, it will freeze really hard, just let set out for a bit before serving!*

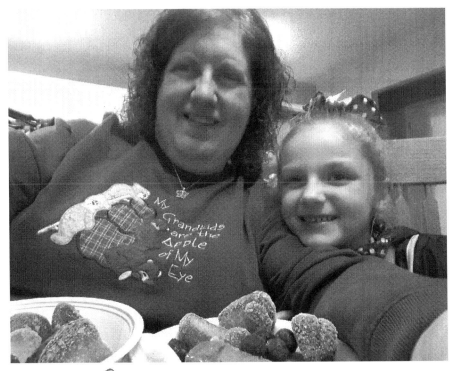

Train to Live . Food is Fuel

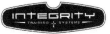

"if you wait for the perfect conditions, you'll never get anything done."

– unknown

Motivation

Sophie's Chocolate Protein Muffins

> 💡 *idea* — A lower sugar option would be to replace maple syrup with Stevia.

2 Ripe Mashed Bananas
2 Eggs
1 cup Natural Peanut, Almond or Cashew Butter
1/2 cup Cocoa Powder
2 scoops Chocolate Egg White or Collagen Powder
1/3 cup Pure Maple Syrup
1 tbsp Alcohol-Free Vanilla
1/2 tsp Baking Soda
1/3 cup Mini Gluten-Free, Dairy-Free Chocolate Chips

Blend all ingredients while leaving chocolate chips aside. Fold chips in when well blended. Bake at 400° for 12 minutes. This recipe can also be used to make cookies as well.

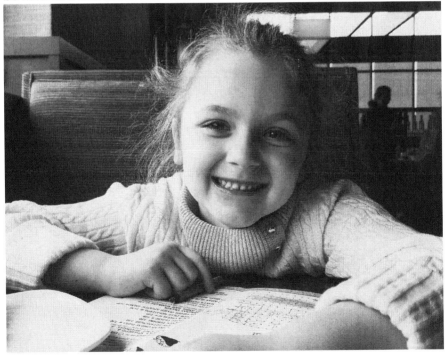

Train to Live . Food is Fuel

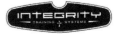

"if you change the way
you look at things, the
things you look at change."

– unknown

Motivation

Sophie's
Cinnamon Roll Protein Muffins

1 cup So Delicious Unsweetened Vanilla Coconut Milk Yogurt
3/4 cup Unsweetened Cinnamon Apple Sauce
1 1/2 cup Gluten-Free Oats
1/2 cup Vanilla Egg White or Collagen Powder
1/3 cup Pure Maple Syrup
2 Eggs
1 tsp Cinnamon
1/2 tsp Alcohol-Free Vanilla
1/4 tsp Sea Salt
1 tsp Aluminum-Free Baking Powder
1/2 cup Unsweetened Golden Raisins

A lower sugar option would be to replace maple syrup with Stevia.

Mix all ingredients in a large bowl or blender. Fold raisins in at the end. Pour into muffin tins. Bake 15 to 20 minutes at 400° or until tooth pick is clean. Sprinkle the top of each one with cinnamon before baking and to place 1 raisin in the center of each one.

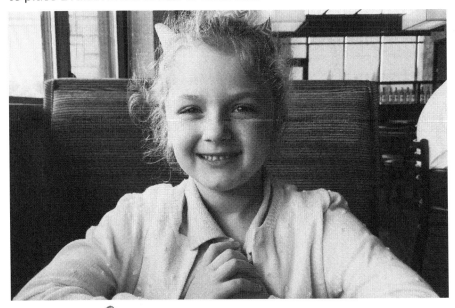

Train to Live . Food is Fuel

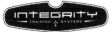

"you are the creator of
your own destiny."

– unknown

Motivation

Sophie's Cinnamon Sugar Shake

1/2 scoop Vanilla Egg White or Collagen Powder
1/2 scoop Cinnamon Apple Ancient Nutrition Bone Broth
      Protein Powder
2 cups Unsweetened Vanilla So Delicious Coconut Milk
1 dash Now Foods Pure Stevia
1/4 tsp Cinnamon

Add all ingredients to your blender, plus ice cubes if preferred. Enjoy!
Also tastes great when you add Unsweetened Vanilla So Delicious Coconut Milk Yogurt to the mix.

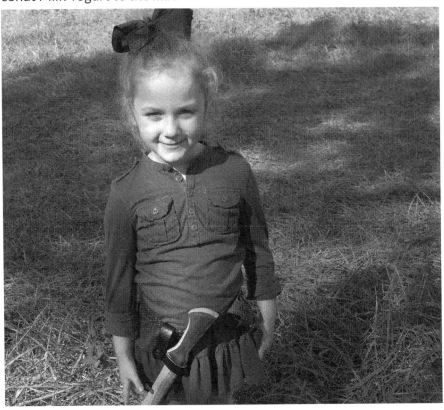

Train to Live · Food is Fuel

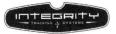

"i'm gonna make the rest of my life, the best of my life."

— Eric Thomas

Motivation

Sophie's
Clean Honey Mustard Dressing

1 Lemon, juiced
1 tbsp Apple Cider Vinegar
1/4 tsp Now Foods Pure Stevia
2 tbsp Dijon Mustard
1/4 tsp Celtic Sea Salt
Pinch of Pepper
1/4 Cup Olive Oil

Blend all ingredients in a blender until well combined. Add to a salad dressing shaker and shake well. Great as a dip and marinade as well.

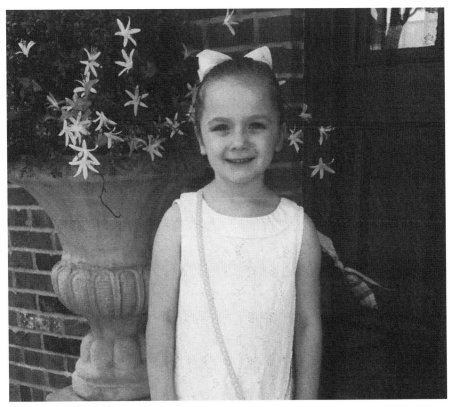

Train to Live . Food is Fuel

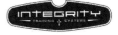

"wow...i really
regretted that workout."

– no one ever

Motivation

Sophie's
Decaf Protein Apple Green Tea

1 Organic Decaf Green Tea Bag
1 Apple Hint Water
2 dashes of Now Foods Pure Stevia
1/2 scoop Vital Proteins Collagen Peptides Unflavored

Add hint water, Stevia and green tea to a large cup or tea pot. Microwave large cup for 2 minutes. Let sit and steep for at least 3 minutes. Drain bag, stir well and add collagen to the tea. A great way to get quality protein. A good way to get antioxidants from the green tea, hydration from the water and 6g of protein from an excellent source.

We use Bigelow decaf green tea bags.

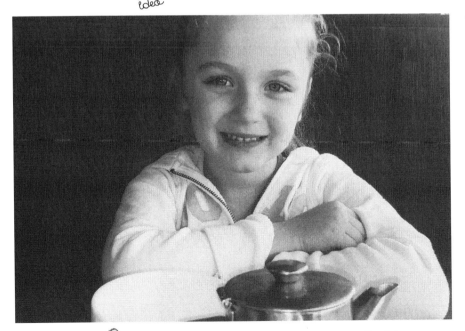

Train to Live . Food is Fuel

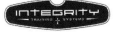

"success isn't always about greatness. it's about consistency. consistent hard work gains success. greatness will come."

- Dwayne "The Rock" Johnson

Motivation

Sophie's First Day of School Fuel

6 slices Uncured Beef Salami (Whole Foods)
1 Organic String Cheese Stick
10 Orange Grape Tomatoes
1/2 cup Blueberries with Stevia
10 Cashews
4 Gluten-Free Crackers
1 Hint Water, any flavor
1 packet Ultima Electrolyte Powder

We have a multi-slot container purchased from Pottery Barn Kids. We keep her lunch in each section. They work great. I add ice, Hint water and her electrolytes to her Thermos. This will help so much with energy and mental clarity.

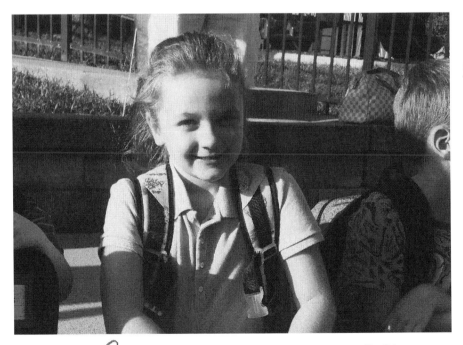

Train to Live . Food is Fuel

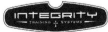

"the body achieves what the mind believes."

— unknown

Motivation

Sophie's
Frogs on a log

Celery
All-Natural Peanut Butter
Golden Raisins

Wash celery and cut into sticks or use the pre-made ones. Spread peanut butter on the celery sticks. Line golden raisins on top of peanut butter! Enjoy! You could also add gluten-free, dairy-free chocolate chips!

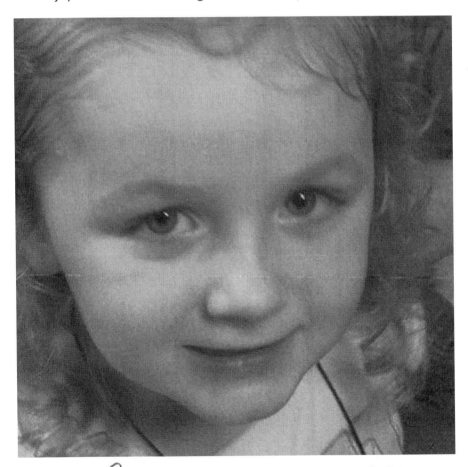

Train to Live . Food is Fuel

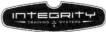

"work hard in silence. let success be your noise."

– Frank Ocean

Motivation

Sophie's Meatloaf Burgers

Burgers
2 lbs of Grass-Fed Ground Beef, *90% lean*
1 bag of Riced Cauliflower
1 tbsp of Debbie's House Seasoning
1 tbsp of Mustard
1 tbsp of Hot Sauce
1/4 cup Minced Onions
1 Onion, chopped in big pieces
2 slices of Turkey Bacon, chopped
  (put off to side)

Sauce
15 oz canned Tomato Sauce
1 1/2 cups of canned Fire-Roasted
  chopped tomatoes with garlic
1/3 cup of Minced Onions
1 1/2 tbsp of Apple Cider Vinegar
2 tbsp of Debbie's House Seasoning
2 tsp of Now Foods Pure Stevia
Pinch of Cayenne Pepper
1 tsp of Black Pepper
1/2 tbsp of Garlic Powder
1 tbsp of Parsley

Preheat oven to 350°. Mix all burger ingredients together in large bowl. Mix all sauce ingredients together, add additional seasoning to taste. Take 1 cup of sauce and add to the hamburger mixture, mixing well. Patty the burgers the same size to keep cooking time consistent throughout, place on metal rack inside of sheet cake pan.
Once pattied, baste each patty with prepared sauce, covering the top of each. Reserve remaining sauce to add to burgers once cooked. Bake for 45 - 55 minutes. After 20 minutes of cooking, add chopped turkey bacon to tops of each burger. Once thoroughly cooked, remove from oven, top with remaining sauce and serve with veggies of choice.

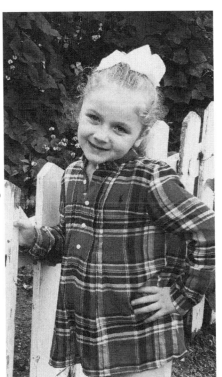

Train to Live . Food is Fuel

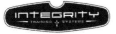

"when you feel like quitting think about why you started."

– unknown

Motivation

Sophie's
Mexican Bacon Burger Wraps

2 lbs of Grass-Fed Ground Beef
2 cans No-Salt Added Organic
    Diced Tomatoes
1 Small Onion, chopped
3/4 cup Organico Bello Organic
    Gluten-Free Marinara Sauce
1 tbsp Frontier Co-Op Mexican
    Fiesta Seasoning
6 slices Sugar-free, Uncured
    Turkey Bacon

1 bag Frozen Riced
    Cauliflower, cooked
1 tbsp Avocado Oil
1 tsp Granulated Garlic
1 tsp Onion Powder
1/2 tbsp Parsley
Salt & Pepper to taste
Home-Style Guacamole
Romaine Lettuce, Butter
Lettuce or Iceberg can be used

Brown ground beef with chopped onion and diced tomatoes. Add Organico Bello marinara sauce to the mixture, continue cooking. In the meantime, place slices of turkey bacon on top of metal rack, placed inside sheet cake pan and bake according to directions. In a separate bowl mix together cooked riced cauliflower, avocado oil, granulated garlic, onion powder, parsley, salt and pepper. Remove bacon from oven and crumble. Remove ground beef mixture from stove. Lay and overlap 2 pieces of lettuce, add 1 heaping spoonful of guacamole to lettuce. Next layer the following: heaping spoonful of ground beef mixture on top of guac, then 1 spoonful of rice mixture on top of that, finish with crumbled bacon. Wrap lettuce like a burrito over mixture and enjoy!

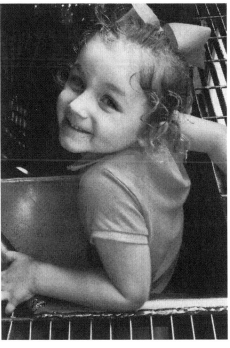

Train to Live . Food is Fuel

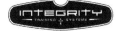

"it comes down to one simple thing: how bad do you want it?"

– unknown

Motivation

Sophie's
Movie Snack Mix

1 cup Banana Chips
1 cup Dried Mango
1 cup Dried Pineapple
1 cup Raw Cashews
1 cup Pistachios
1 cup Raw Almonds

Combine all ingredients together. Create snack bags for your purse. Avoid that GMO filled popcorn. Keep your kids healthy!

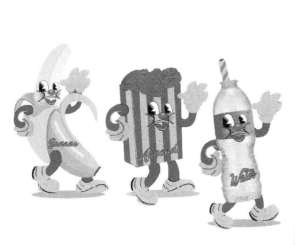

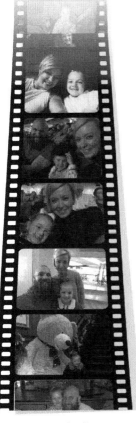

Train to Live . Food is Fuel

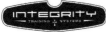

"don't count the days,

make the days count."

- Muhammad Ali

Motivation

Sophie's
Mustard Dill Salmon

(4) 5 oz. servings of Salmon
3 tbsp Fresh Lemon Juice
1 tbsp White Wine Vinegar
1/4 cup Extra-Virgin Olive Oil
1/2 tsp Dried Dill
1/8 tsp Salt, to taste
1/8 tsp Black Pepper, to taste
1/2 tbsp Dijion Mustard

In a small bowl, whisk all the ingredients together until emulsified. Taste for salt/pepper, add more if needed. Cover and refrigerate until ready to use. Shake well before using. Pour over salmon. Bake in over on 350° for 30 minutes or until desired doneness.

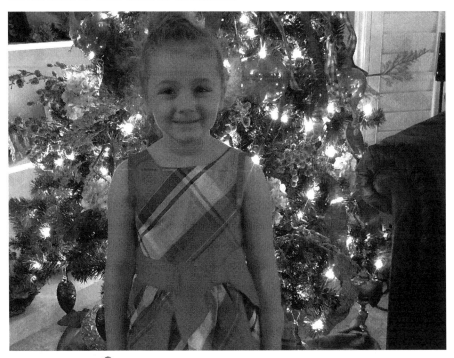

Train to Live . Food is Fuel

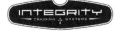

"obstacles can't stop you.

problems can't stop you.

people can't stop you.

only you can stop you."

— unknown

Motivation

Sophie's Peanut Butter Protein Cookies

1 cup of Smuckers All-Natural Peanut Butter
1/2 cup Baking Stevia
1 whole large Egg
1 tsp Alcohol-Free Vanilla
1 tsp Aluminum-Free Baking Powder
1 tsp Cinnamon
1 tbsp Vanilla Jay Robb's Protein Powder
1 whole Mashed Banana
1 tbsp Agave

Combine all ingredients into a large bowl. Mix with whisk or hand mixer until well blended. Use small ice cream scoop to spread evenly distributed cookies across parchment paper or lined cookie sheet. Cook on 350° for 10-12 minutes. Should make 16 bite size cookies.

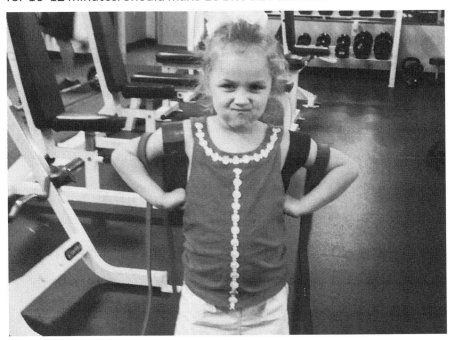

Train to Live . Food is Fuel

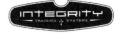

"believe in yourself and all that you are. know that there is something inside of you that is greater than any obstacle."

– unknown

Motivation

Sophie's
Oven-Dried Strawberries

1 lb Strawberries (washed and dried)

Preheat oven to 200 °. Slice strawberries into uniform slices, approximately 1/8 inch thick. *Note: if you slice the strawberries thicker, it will take longer for them to dry.* Arrange strawberries on parchment or silicone baking liner, leaving space between each slice. Bake in oven for approximately 2 hours, until tops are dry. Flip strawberries over so and bake for another hour or so until fully dehydrated. Once cool, store in an airtight container at room temperature. The dried strawberries can be stored for several months at room temp without spoiling.

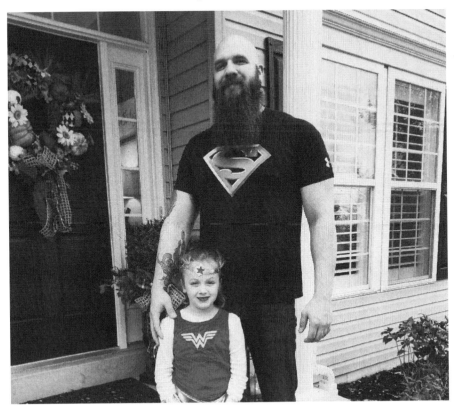

Train to Live . Food is Fuel

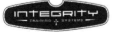

"the hard part isn't getting your body in shape. the hard part is getting your mind in shape."

– unknown

Motivation

Sophie's
Power Protein Muffins

A lower sugar option would be to replace maple syrup with Stevia.

idea

1 Mashed Ripe Banana
2 1/4 cups Gluten-Free Oats
1/4 cup Pure Maple Syrup
1 1/2 scoops Chocolate Egg White Protein Powder
1/3 cup Natural Peanut Butter
1 Egg
1 cup Vanilla Unsweetened Coconut Milk
1/2 tsp Cinnamon
1/4 tsp Salt
1 tsp Baking Powder
1 tsp Alcohol-Free Vanilla
1/2 cup Gluten-Free Dairy Free Chocolate Chips

Blend all ingredients together well, leaving chocolate chips aside. Fold chips in. Spread into greased muffin pan. Cook at 350° for 25-30 minutes. Store in airtight container after cooled, in fridge, and warm up prior to serving.

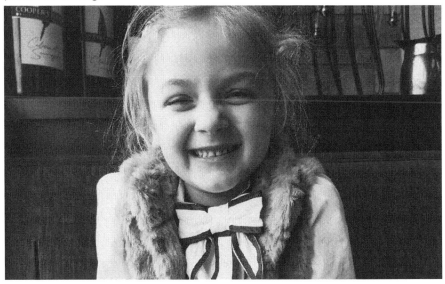

Train to Live . Food is Fuel

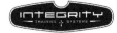

"i may not be there yet,

but i'm closer than

i was yesterday."

– unknown

Motivation

Sophie's
Protein Energy Balls

1/2 cup Natural Peanut, Almond or Cashew Butter
1 cup Gluten-Free Oats
1/3 cup Pure Maple Syrup
1 tsp Alcohol-Free Vanilla
1/2 tsp Cinnamon
1/2 cup Ground Flax Meal
2 tbsp Chocolate Egg White or Collagen Powder
1/3 cup Unsweetened Golden Raisins
6 tbsp Gluten and Dairy-FreeChocolate Chips

Mix all ingredients together well in a large bowl. Roll into balls. Place in an air tonight container. Keep in fridge or freezer.

A lower sugar option would be to replace maple syrup with Stevia.

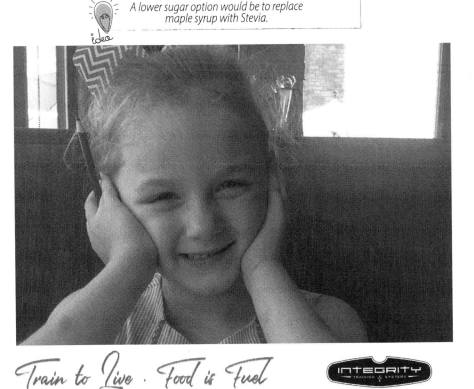

Train to Live . Food is Fuel

INTEGRITY

"don't be afraid of being a beginner."

– unknown

Motivation

Sophie's
Protein Peach Popsicles

3 Fresh Peaches, chopped without skin
1 Peach Hint Water
3 pinches of Now Foods Stevia
1 scoop Vital Proteins Collagen Peptides Unflavored

Add all items into a blender. Blend well until fully combined and completely liquid. Pour into Popsicle molds. Freeze for 30 minutes. Enjoy!

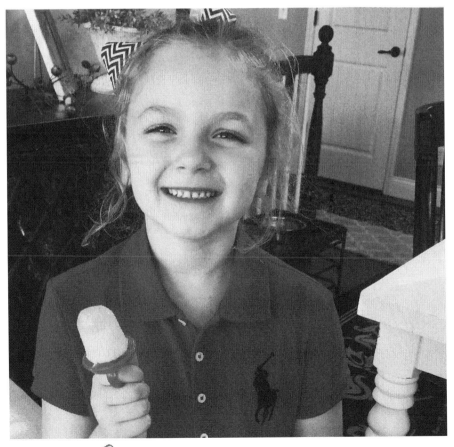

Train to Live . Food is Fuel

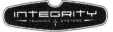

"70% of people that start
a fitness plan quit.

except you.

not this time."

— unknown

Motivation

Sophie's
Pumpkin Apple Protein Muffins

1/2 cup Natural Almond, Cashew or Peanut Butter
1/2 cup Gluten-Free Oats
1 Egg
1/2 cup Pumpkin
1 Mashed Banana
1/4 cup Pure Maple Syrup
2 scoops Vanilla Egg White or Collagen Powder
1/2 tsp Aluminum-Free Baking Powder
1/2 tsp Cinnamon
1/2 tsp Alcohol-Free Vanilla
1/4 tsp Sea Salt
1 dash Pumpkin Pie Spice
1/2 cup Apple, chopped and
    peeled
1/3 cup Unsweetened Golden
    Raisins

idea   *A lower sugar option would be to replace maple syrup with Stevia.*

Blend all ingredients together well, leaving apple and raisins aside. Fold in apple and raisins after blended. Pour into muffin tins. Bake at 350° for 20 to 25 minutes or until golden brown.

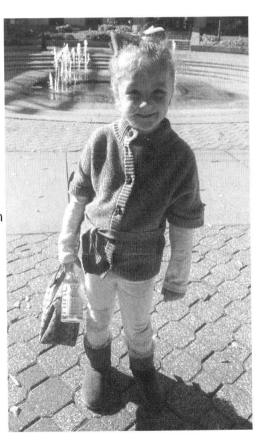

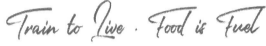

Train to Live . Food is Fuel

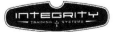

"you've only got 3 choices in life: give up, give in, or give it all you've got."

– unknown

Motivation

Sophie's
Pumpkin Yogurt Parfait

1 1/2 cup Unsweetened Vanilla So Delicious Coconut Milk Yogurt
1/2 cup Pumpkin Puree
1/2 tsp Cinnamon
1/2 tsp Alcohol-Free Vanilla
1/2 scoop Apple Cinnamon Ancient Nutrition Bone Broth
        Protein Powder
1/2 scoop Vanilla Egg White or Collagen Powder
1 dash Now Foods Pure Stevia Powder
1 Gluten-Free Graham Cracker

Combine all ingredients into your blender, blend until well combined.
Place graham cracker into a Ziploc bag and crumble. Pour onto the top
of the yogurt. Enjoy!

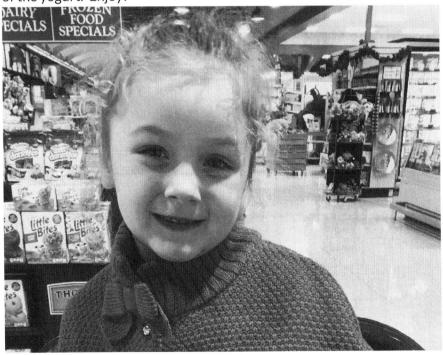

Train to Live . Food is Fuel

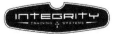

"when you really want something, you will find a way. when you don't really want something, you'll find an excuse.."

– unknown

Motivation

Sophie's
Roasted Brussels Sprouts

2 - 3 lbs. of Fresh Brussels Sprouts (cut in half)
1 large Shallot
1 tbsp Olive Oil
Sea Salt
Pepper
1 tbsp of Onion Powder
2 Cloves of Garlic, minced

Sauté shallot, garlic and olive oil. Roll fresh brussels sprouts in the mixture. Foil line a sheet cake pan, lay veggie mixture out evenly. Bake at 350° for 30 minutes, toss them around and cook 15 minutes more, or until desired doneness.

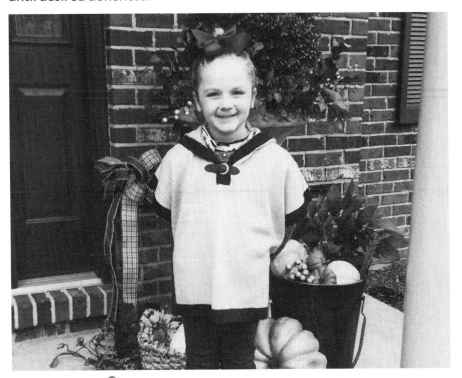

Train to Live . Food is Fuel

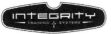

"there is no diet that will

do what eating

healthy does."

– unknown

Motivation

Sophie's Salami Roll-Ups

4 pieces of Uncured Beef Salami (Whole Foods)
1/2 piece of String Cheese cut down the middle
3 Hamburger Dill Pickles

Set 2 pieces of salami overlapping each other by 1/4. Using a paper towel, pat dry the pickles well and center on the salami slices. Lay the cheese on top of the pickles. Roll it all up and stick a tooth pick down the center. Serve!

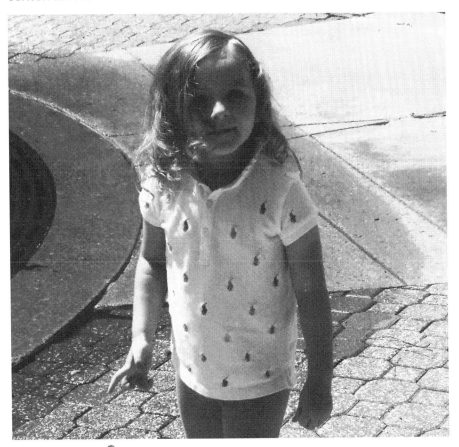

Train to Live . Food is Fuel

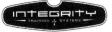

"it always seems impossible until it's done."

– unknown

Motivation

Sophie's
Shallot Vinaigrette

2 tbsp Shallot, minced
2 tsp Garlic, minced
2 tbsp Red Wine Vinegar
1/3 cup Olive Oil
1 tsp Sea Salt
1/2 tsp Pepper

Whisk all together to create an excellent dressing for a salad or marinade for meat.

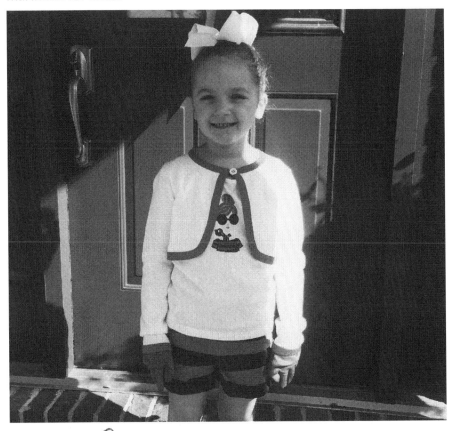

Train to Live · Food is Fuel

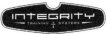

"every accomplishment
starts with the
decision to try."

– unknown

Motivation

Sophie's Shopping Day Snack Bag

1 cup Green or Black Olives
1/2 cup Orange Grape Tomatoes
1/2 cup Red Grape Tomatoes
1 cup Carrots, chopped dime size
1 Organic String Cheese, chopped dime size

Towel dry the olives well. Combine all ingredients into one large Ziploc bag. A great source of fat and carbs. Great when combined with the protein green tea.

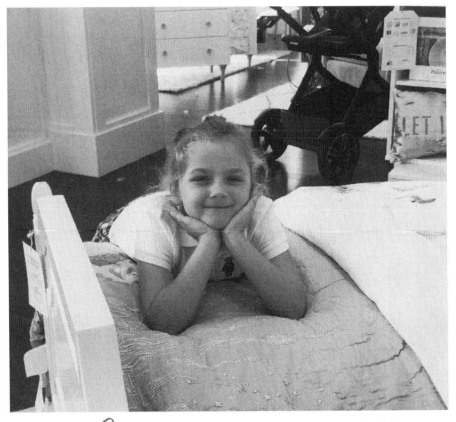

Train to Live . Food is Fuel

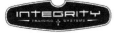

"don't give up what you want most for what you want now."

– unknown

Motivation

Sophie's
Slushies

Celestial Seasonings Herbal Caffeine-Free Tea
- Country Peach Passion
- Blueberry
- Black Cherry Berry

Any Flavor Hint Water

For Tea: Heat 1 or 2 cups of water in the microwave for 90 seconds. Put a teabag in each cup of water, steep for a little while, then chill in the fridge. After It's chilled, fill ice cube trays with the tea, keep a little of the liquid tea in the fridge. When frozen, put cubes in a Ninja or blender & crush. Put in a cup & add a little of the liquid tea to make the slushie! Hint Water: Just pour in ice cube trays and freeze. Save a little hint water for the slushie. Sophie & I like ours unsweetened, but you can add stevia if you prefer a sweet taste!

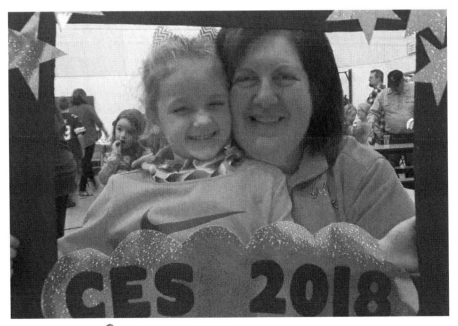

Train to Live . Food is Fuel

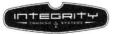

"change happens when the pain of staying the same is greater than the pain of change."

– unknown

Motivation

Sophie's
Spaghetti

1-1 ¹/² lbs Grass-Fed Beef or Ground Round Beef
1-1 ¹/² jars of your choice of Low-Sugar Organic Marinara Sauce
Frozen Riced Cauliflower
Garlic Powder
Onion Powder
Pink Himalayan Salt

Brown ground beef in a wok type skillet or pot, season with garlic powder, onion powder and salt and cook until browned. Drain off any excess grease. *Note: I rinse the ground beef with very hot water also, then add more garlic & onion powder & salt!* Put beef back into pan, add the marinara sauce, let simmer on med/low for a bit. Heat riced cauliflower in microwave long enough to thaw, then put it a bowl with lid, season with garlic powder, onion powder & salt. Stir & heat up thoroughly. Serve riced cauliflower on plate topped with meat marinara sauce. Sophie likes it with brussels sprouts & green beans for sides.

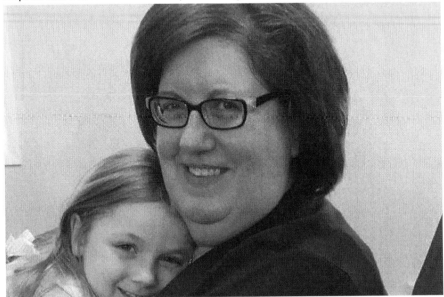

Train to Live . Food is Fuel

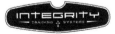

"being challenged in life is
inevitable. being
defeated is optional."

– unknown

Motivation

Sophie's Strawberry Pineapple Protein Popsicles

1 cup Pineapple, cubed
1 cup Strawberries, chopped
1 Pineapple Hint Water
2 pinches of Now Foods Pure Stevia Powder
1 scoop Vital Proteins Collagen Peptides Unflavored

Blend all ingredients well until liquid. Pour into Popsicle molds. Freeze for 30 minutes. Enjoy!

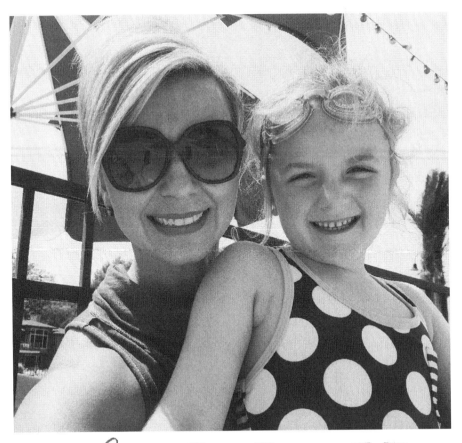

Train to Live . Food is Fuel

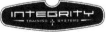

"action always
beats intention."

– unknown

Motivation

Sophie's
Strawberry Power Yogurt

1 cup Unsweetened Vanilla So Delicious Coconut Milk Yogurt
1/2 cup Strawberries, chopped
1/2 scoop Strawberry Jay Robb's Egg White Protein Powder
1 tbsp Strawberry-Banana Barlean's Flax Seed Oil
1 dash of Now Foods Pure Stevia Powder

Blend all ingredients in your blender. I like to use frozen berries that are thawed that create a juice. These are also great frozen in Popsicle molds.

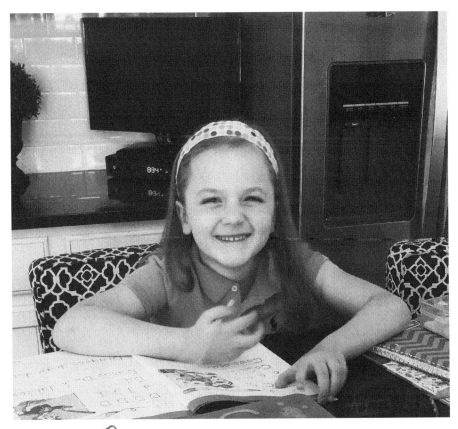

Train to Live . Food is Fuel

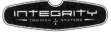

"being defeated is often a temporary condition ... giving up is what makes it permanent."

– unknown

Motivation

Sophie's Strawberry Protein Muffins

> 💡 *A lower sugar option would be to replace maple syrup with Stevia.*

1/2 cup So Delicious Unsweetened Vanilla Coconut Milk Yogurt
1/2 cup Unsweetened Applesauce
2 cups Gluten-Free Oats
2 scoops Vanilla Egg White or Collagen Powder
1/3 cup Pure Maple Syrup
2 Eggs
1 tsp Alcohol-Free Vanilla
1/4 tsp Salt
1 tsp Aluminum-Free Baking Powder
1 cup Strawberries, chopped
2 tbsp Strawberry All-Fruit Preserves
1 tsp Cinnamon

Mix all ingredients in a larger bowl with mixer or blender. Fold strawberries in at the end. Pour into muffin tins. Bake 30 minutes at 350° or until tooth pick comes out clean. Place a sliver of strawberry on the top of each one.

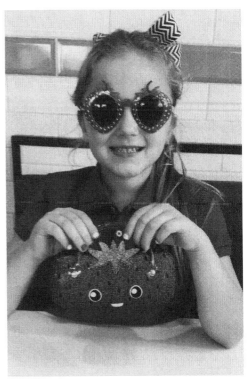

Train to Live · Food is Fuel

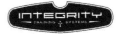

"fit is not a destination, it is a way of life."

– unknown

Motivation

Sophie's
Sweet Apple Sauté

4 Pink Lady Apples, chopped
2 tsp Cinnamon
1 tsp Now Foods Pure Stevia
2 tbsp Avocado Oil
1 tsp Alcohol-Free Vanilla

Sauté all ingredients on low to medium temperature. Tastes best when you slow cook them. Serves great with sweet vinaigrette chicken strips.

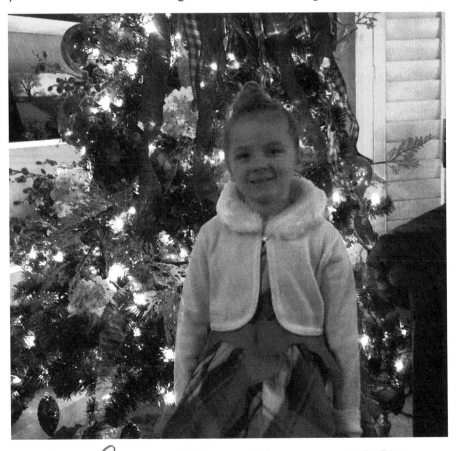

Train to Live · Food is Fuel

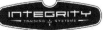

"training gives us an outlet for suppressed energies created by stress and thus tones the spirit just as exercise conditions the body."

- Arnold Schwarzenegger

Motivation

Sophie's
Sweet Potato Fries

1 medium sized Sweet Potato, peeled
1 tbsp Avocado Oil
1 tsp Debbie's House Seasoning

Slice the potato into sticks thin enough to bake evenly. Try to keep the fries the same size. Place a cooling rack inside a sheet cake pan. Drizzle oil on potato in a bowl. Add seasoning. Spread evenly on cooking rack. Bake at 400 ° for 10 minutes. Flip each fry and cook for 10 more minutes or until desired doneness. We eat this with a grilled chicken breast after dance each Wednesday.

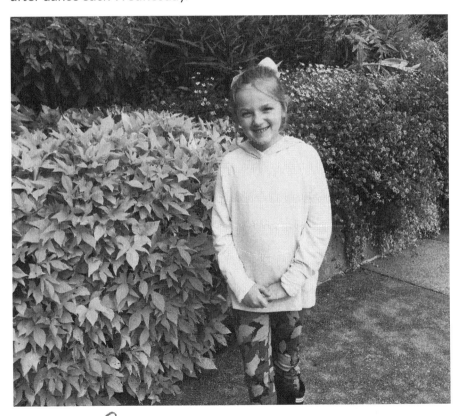

Train to Live . Food is Fuel

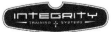

"your health is an investment, not an expense."

– unknown

Motivation

Sophie's
Sweet Vinaigrette Chicken

8 Bare Chicken Tenderloins
1 bottle Sweet Vinaigrette Simple Girl
2 tbsp Avocado Oil
Salt & Pepper to taste

Marinate chicken overnight in half bottle of dressing. Warm oil in a grill pan. Pan sear each side until browned well. Set chicken on a cooling rack inside a sheet cake pan. Bake chicken on 350° for another 10-15 minutes until done inside. Great when coupled with bacon and avocado mayo for a lettuce wrap. Also good when dipped into my Clean Honey Mustard Dressing recipe.

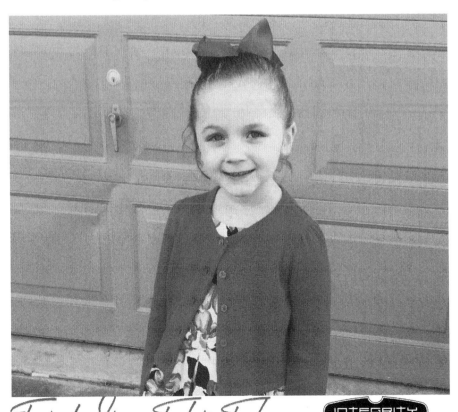

Train to Live · Food is Fuel

INTEGRITY
TRAINING SYSTEMS

"i believe that the greatest gift you can give your family and the world is a healthy you."

- Joyce Meyer

Motivation

Taylor's Easy Egg Omelet Muffins

Great for entertaining guests or meal prep

12 Eggs
1 cup of Fresh Spinach
1 large Tomato (diced), or 3/4 cup of Cherry Tomatoes, quartered
1/2 cup Bell pepper, diced
1/2 cup Onion, diced
Salt and Pepper to taste
Salsa (*optional*)
Avocado (*optional*)

Note: sub out any ingredients to make your favorite omelet!

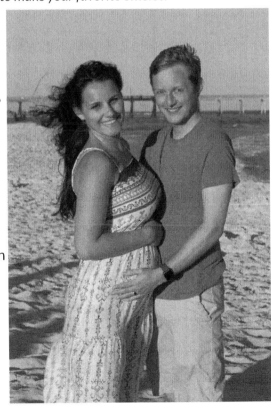

Preheat oven to 350°.
Grease down muffin pan. In
a large bowl, combine eggs,
spinach, tomatoes, peppers,
and onions (or your choice
of any other ingredients).
Divide evenly into muffin
pan place in oven for 20-25
mins. Let cool. To remove,
run knife around edges.
Serve topped with fresh
avocado and salsa or keep in
fridge for up to 3 days.

Train to Live . Food is Fuel

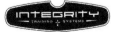

"it never gets easier, you just get better."

– unknown

Motivation

Taylor's
Roasted Tomato & Garlic Marinara Sauce

4 large Tomatoes
6-8 Cloves of Garlic (*the more the better!*)
Fresh Basil Leaves
1 tsp of Apple Cider Vinegar (*optional*)
Olive Oil or Avocado Oil
Salt and Pepper, to taste

Preheat over to 400°. Place tomatoes and garlic on foiled cookie sheet. Drizzle olive or avocado oil over tomatoes and garlic. Bake for 1 hour or until brown. Let stand and cool, then peel skins off tomatoes. Place in blender or food processor with basil, salt, pepper, and vinegar. Blend. Pour over zucchini noodles or Spaghetti squash and serve. Or save in fridge for up to four days. *Makes 2-3 cups*

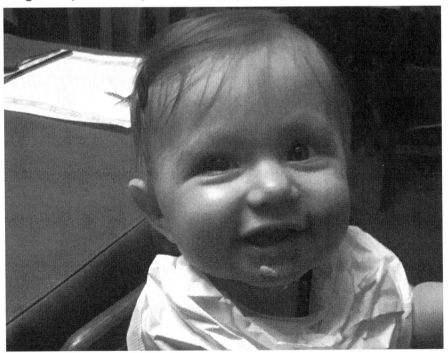

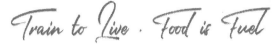
Train to Live . Food is Fuel

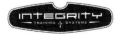
INTEGRITY
TRAINING SYSTEMS

"at first they'll ask you why you're doing it. then they'll ask you how you did it."

– unknown

Motivation

Taylor's
Turkey Meatloaf Cupcakes
Amazing for large crowds or meal prep

1/2 large Onion, chopped
1 Bell Pepper, seeds and stem removed, chopped
1 Jalapeño, seeds and stem removed, chopped (*optional*)
1/2 cup of Instant Oats
1/2 tsp Cumin
1/4 tsp Paprika
1 tsp Dried Oregano
2 tsp Garlic Powder
1 tbsp Olive Oil
2 Eggs
20 oz Ground Turkey Meat
Salt and Pepper to taste

Preheat oven to 375°. Grease muffin pan. Mix all ingredients together. Don't be afraid to get your hands dirty! Roll into balls and place into muffin pan. Place into oven for 30-35 mins. To remove, use knife along the edges. Serve warm or save for meet prep.
Cook time: 35 mins | Yields 12 cupcakes

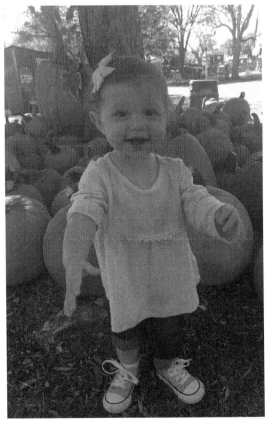

Train to Live . Food is Fuel

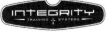

"it's easier to wake up early and work out than it is to look in the mirror each day and not like what you see."

– unknown

Motivation

The Summers's
Best Steak You've Ever Had
- trust me

Steak
4 (12 oz) Rib-Eye Steaks, 1 ¹/⁴" thick, at room temperature
4 tbsp Olive Oil
Kosher Salt and Freshly Ground Black Pepper, to taste

Garlic Compound Butter
1/2 cup Kirkland's Unsalted Butter, at room temperature
1/4 cup Fresh Parsley Leaves, chopped
3 Cloves Garlic, minced
Zest of 1 lemon
1 tsp Basil, chopped
1/2 tsp Kosher Salt
1/4 tsp Ground Black Pepper
pinch of Cayenne Pepper

Garlic compound butter: Combine butter, parsley, garlic, lemon zest, basil, salt, pepper and cayenne pepper in a medium bowl. Transfer mixture to parchment paper; shape into a log. Roll in parchment to 1 ¹/² inches in diameter, twisting the ends to close. Refrigerate until ready to use, up to 1 week.*

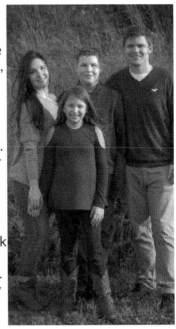

Preheat oven to broil. Place an oven-proof skillet in the oven. Using paper towels, pat both sides of the steak dry. Drizzle with olive oil; season with salt and pepper, to taste. Remove skillet from the oven and heat over medium-high heat. Place the steak in the middle of the skillet and cook until a dark crust has formed, about 1 minute. Using tongs, flip, and cook for an additional 60 seconds. Place skillet into the oven and cook until desired doneness is reached, about 4-5 minutes for medium-rare, flipping once. Let rest for 3-5 minutes. Serve immediately with garlic compound butter.

Train to Live . Food is Fuel

"our greatest weakness and greatest power lies within our mindset."

– unknown

Motivation

The Summers's
Gummy Bears

(2) 20g boxes of Simply The Best All-Natural Jel Dessert, any flavor
   (*I have only been able to find these online, but they are worth the search*)
1/4 cup Vital Proteins Beef Gelatin Unflavored
1/2 cup of <u>Cold</u> Water

I found silicone unicorn and bear molds at Micheal's. You can also find some on Amazon.
Place the cold water in a small saucepan that has not been on the heat yet. Sprinkle the unflavored gelatin into the water and lightly whisk. Allow the gelatin to bloom for a minute or two and then add in the flavored jel. Slowly heat the mixture over medium low heat, whisking often until the jel is completely dissolved. It should be a smooth liquid mixture now, not gritty. Remove from heat and pour into glass measuring cup so that you can pour into molds. Place in the refrigerator or at least 30 minutes. Pop out and enjoy!

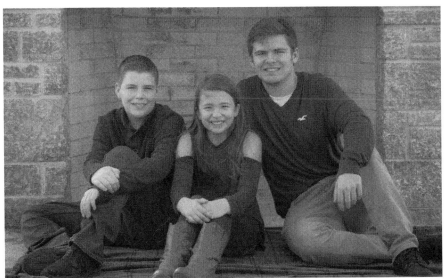

Train to Live . Food is Fuel

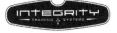

"our strength grows out of

our weaknesses."

– unknown

Motivation

The Summers's
Sugar-Free Candied Pecans

2 1/2 cups Pecans, or Nuts of choice
1 Egg White
1/2 cup Swerve Granular
1 1/2 tsp Cinnamon
1/8 tsp Salt

Preheat oven to 300°. Line a 15"x10"x1" pan with foil and spray with cooking oil. Place nuts in a bowl and stir if not already mixed. Beat egg white in a separate bowl until foamy and stir into the nuts until evenly coated. In another bowl, mix the Swerve, cinnamon, and salt and pour over the nuts. Stir until evenly coated, then scoop onto the baking sheet, using a spoon or fingers to get the nuts in a single layer. Bake for 12-18 minutes, stirring every four minutes, until toasted. There's a fine line between thoroughly cooked and burnt, keep checking on them. Allow to cool on wax paper and store in an airtight container. When serving, get a small amount for yourself, then have someone hide the whole container because you will eat them all...in one sitting...

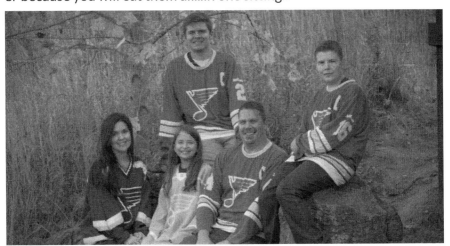

Train to Live · Food is Fuel

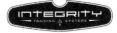

"turn a setback into a

comeback."

– unknown

Motivation

The Yuppy Puppy's Grain Free Peanut Butter Dog Treats

1 medium Banana
2 large Eggs
1/2 cup Creamy Peanut Butter
1 cup Chickpea Flour
1/2 cup Coconut Flour
1/4 tsp Baking Soda
Dog Bone Cookie Cutter (or any cookie cutter)

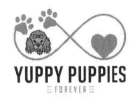

YUPPY PUPPIES
≡ FOREVER ≡

Preheat oven to 350 °. In a large bowl, mash banana until smooth. Beat in eggs until fully mixed, then beat in peanut butter until smooth. Once smooth, fold in chickpea flour, coconut flour and baking soda with spatula. Knead with hands until all flour has been folded into the dough. Once dough is kneaded, roll out onto a parchment surface until dough is $^{1/4}$" thick. (Additional flour may be needed here.) Using your dog bone cookie cutter (or whatever cookie cutter you decide to use) cut out and place on baking sheet. Bake for 14 minutes, or until golden brown. Let cool completely before serving to your pooch or packing/storing!
Servings: Approx. 24 treats

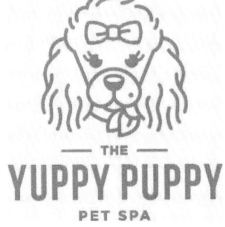

— THE —
YUPPY PUPPY
PET SPA

Train to live . Food is Fuel

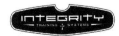

Thank you to an amazing staff and trainers. You are champions. God bless you for supporting the vision I have to bless people and save people through health and wellness.

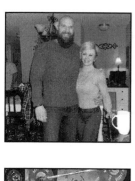
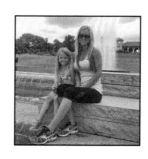
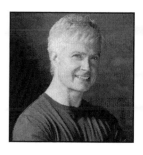

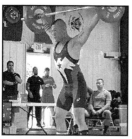
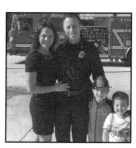
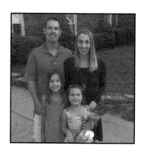

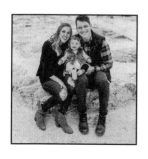

I can do all things through Christ who strengthens me.
Philippians 4:13

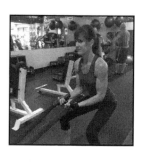

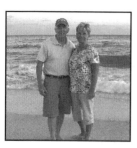
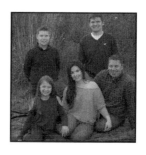
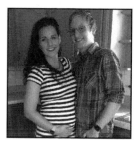

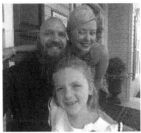
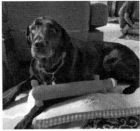
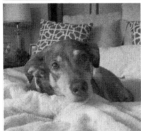
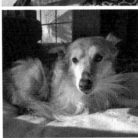

Dr. Anna Bone
(314) 961-1807

Dr. Bligh
www.drblighmd.com

Dr. Ava Frick, Pet Rehab & Pain Clinic
www.AnimalRehabStlouis.com

Dr. Ian McDonald
www.cmbchiro.com

Foxhole Partners
www.foxholepartners.wordpress.com

Integrity Training Systems
www.integritytraininggroup.com

O'fallon Nutrition
www.ofallonnutrition.com

Pure Plates
www.pureplatesstl.com

Yuppy Puppy Pet Spa
www.yuppypuppyspa.com

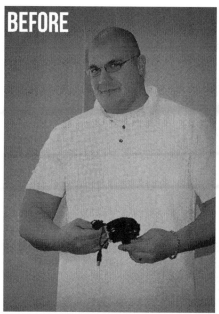
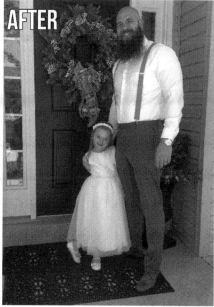
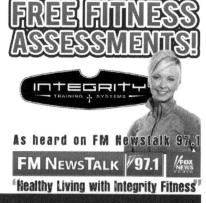

Made in the USA
Columbia, SC
25 September 2022

67589821R00091